Liz
I am so
thankful
here to'b
my gowl' Enjoy

Essentially Better
essential oils for
people with feelings

Wendy Bruton, Ph.D.

Essentially Better
Essential Oils for People with Feelings
By Wendy Bruton, PhD

ISBN: 1984034529
ISBN-13: 978-1984034526

DEDICATION

TO LOGAHN, CONRAD, MALIKAI, AND AVERIE. I'M SO GLAD THAT I GET TO BE YOUR GRAMMY!

ACKNOWLEDGMENTS

Thank you to:

My husband *Scott*. Thank you for supporting everything I do, no matter how crazy it seems! You make me believe I can do anything. I love doing life with you.

Sue Stratton. I blame you. I love you. Thanks for sharing essential oils with me, and for dragging me kicking and screaming into this business! I am so very thankful.

Lisa & Jeanette. Thank you for being my BFF's. Thank you for spending a whole weekend at the beach reading and editing this book. I could not do life without you!

Sarah, Kiara, Allison and Jenny. I am so thankful to be doing this with my girls. I love being your mom! I am unbelievably proud of the women you are. You make this adventure perfect!

CONTENTS

OBLIGATORY DISCLAIMER

I am a licensed professional counselor. I have a PhD in Counseling and Counselor Education. I have education and credentialing which gives me the authority to diagnose mental health disorders, and to teach therapists about diagnosis. However, I am not credentialed to train others to treat mental health diagnoses with Essential Oils.

Please hear me... this is important. I am in no way asserting that essential oils can cure mental health disorders. For that matter, neither can pharmaceuticals. My only intention is to provide a place where people can learn about different symptoms and behaviors which may be part of a mental health diagnosis, and to list essential oils that have been shown to support wellness within those areas.

Part 1

Essential Oils for People with Feelings

CHAPTER 1
THE NEW ME

Writing always makes me question myself. I am not sure where to start, or how to eloquently say all of the seemingly important things running around in my head. The conversation I had at lunch the other day made those questioning voices in my head even louder. "This isn't you. I mean, you can do whatever you want, but this essential oil thing really doesn't seem like you." Jeanette was right. She has been one of my best friends for over 20 years, she knows me better than most people in the world, and she was right.

This is not me. This is not who I am, or at least who I have been. I mean, I am a Doctor for goodness sake. I am smart, really smart. I am successful. I have a strong reputation. I am skeptical. I need proof. I have a thriving practice, great friends, and a supportive family. What am I thinking? I am not the kind of person who does classes on essential oils, and I sure don't spend time writing a book about them. I am on a career path that many people envy. I don't "jump on bandwagons." I am a researcher. It takes a long time for me to believe in new ideas, and even then more reluctantly. This is not me...or at least it hasn't been until now.

The first time I allowed myself to entertain the idea that essential oils might benefit mental health, was when I was working in a hospital emergency room. I evaluated patients in order to determine if they should be admitted to the hospital for mental health issues. One night I was in a patient's room with a Psychiatrist on staff. The patient was refusing to take medications. The side effects had been horrible in the past so she was not willing to fill any prescription. The doctor started talking to her and her family about essential oils. He said they would work very effectively over time if she would be consistent in using them. Then he wrote her a prescription for essential oils. I had no idea at that point what essential oils could do, not even a clue. I didn't know how or why they worked. But this physician who was able to prescribe pharmaceuticals had just written a prescription for an essential oil. I took notice.

I got my *Young Living Premium Starter Kit* at a class my friend from church held at her house. I had just opened a new counseling center that was promoting a holistic approach to mental health. But my definition of holistic only included anything that had a lot of research behind it. The "woo-woo" didn't fit into my version of holistic. We had yoga, massage, hypnotherapy, and great mental health therapists. I got the essential oils to make the office smell nice, more of a spa-like environment. I still didn't see them as therapeutic, or understand that they could be a potential resource for helping the overall wellness of our clients.

One day I came across some research completely by accident. I started to pay attention. These smart, well educated people were using essential oils to help with things like emotional regulation, supporting sleep rhythms, and making it possible for people to tolerate distress in effective ways. Along with many other physical issues, essential oils were making an impact on mental health. I was finding myself quite intrigued.

A friend of mine was given a book written by someone who was using essential oils in counseling. She gave it to me and I read it. I actually wasn't sure I was going to like the book. But as I read through it my interest got peeked. The author, a Psychologist, described significant breakthroughs that he had seen with his patients. These essential oils were supporting the healing process of people with profound trauma.

I began talking about what I was reading with the team of therapists at my counseling center. They each began doing their own research and we all began using specific essential oils in our counseling sessions. Almost immediately we started to see a change. People started asking how to get these oils. They started coming to the classes we were giving on how to use essential oils for emotional regulation. Soon my center became a vendor for *Young Living Essential Oils*. People were feeling better. They noticed a difference when they were in the office while the oils were being diffused. They were having breakthroughs in counseling that both the client and the counselor were attributing to the use of oils. I became a believer.

My husband and I began using oils more and more in our own lives. We saw a difference in our health, our sleep, and our mood. I realized that my life, both personally and professionally, had been changed by the use of these natural products. Of course it was. God has given us all we need to move toward physical, emotional, and spiritual wellness.

I am confident that this is where I am supposed to be. I am excited about this book and the potential it has to help people who are struggling with mental health issues. I am excited to help moms, dads, sisters, brothers, friends, and employers who have people in their lives struggling to just be okay. I know this information can be life changing. I have seen it.

I have gone to school for a long time. I have a Bachelor's Degree in Social Work, a Master's Degree in Counseling, and a PhD in Counseling Education. I have a lot of information that would be helpful to people who are struggling with emotional unrest. But this is the first thing I wanted to write a book about. Essential Oils can help. They help people move toward wellness in a way that makes it easier to speed up the process. Essential oils are natural, made by God to help your mind, body, and soul heal. This is worth my time.

If you are looking for an academic book on oils and the science behind them, this is not that book. I will direct you to many resources where you can find that information. This book is intended to be a conversation about mental health and how you can use essential oils to help you move toward wellness. I hope it is helpful and supportive! I'm so glad you are on this journey with me.

CHAPTER 2
EMOTIONS: THE GOOD, BAD, & UGLY

"Sometimes feelings suck." One of my clients said this to me the other day and I had to completely agree. Most of the time I would rather think my way through hard situations then to feel my way through them. It's hard, painful, and time consuming. But feelings are part of our makeup... they come from our biology. Much of the time our feelings come from our chemistry... not our character. They are a product of brain chemistry. We feel what our brain and body want us to feel. There is purpose for our feelings, no matter how much they suck!

What are emotions anyway?

We live in a very complex world. Our brains and bodies are not able to take in all that is happening around us. At any given moment there are trillions of pieces of information about the world around us that are bombarding our senses. Our brains work hard to select a small amount of input that it can process at any given time. When things happen to change what information is familiar to us it causes a biological response that creates what we experience as emotion.

"Changes in states like pain, pleasure, hunger, thirst, body temperature, and respiratory rate trigger emotions. Humans are more sensitive to changes in sound and scent than to visual patterns, and more emotionally responsive to pain and thirst than pleasure and hunger. In general, we respond with more intense emotion to changes we hear and smell than to those we see and to those that hurt and parch more than pleasures and appetites." ~Steven Stosny, PhD (from "The Function of Emotion" published in Psychology Today, 2016)

Sometimes emotions are triggered by stimuli outside the body, and sometimes they are triggered by the things that happen inside our minds like memories, thoughts, or other emotions. Either way, emotions produce an unlimited amount of changes in our bodies. There are changes in our heart rate, muscle tone, energy level, tone of our voice, body posture, and facial expressions. These chemical changes in our brain that we experience as emotion, signal organs in our body to speed up or slow down. They have the power to increase or decrease our breathing, heart rate, and even the rate in which we are able to make decisions. Emotions are able to increase our ability to think clearly, or completely distort and disrupt our ability to mentally process anything that comes our way. We all have experience with this. When we are excited about doing something creative and fun, our minds feel like they open up and ideas can keep flowing. However, when we feel things like shame, hopelessness, or a sense of profound sadness, our brains and bodies can simply shut down. We feel slow, lethargic, frozen, or ready to run away.

Why on Earth do we have feelings?

Feelings make us feel alive and experience the world.

To talk about emotions, we first need to talk about memory. In order to create a memory, our brains need both an event and an emotion. These then are filed together in our brain to create a memory. So many things happen to us each moment of our lives that we would not have room to store all of them. In order to recall memories, our brains were created to need both the event, and an emotion attached to it. The bigger the event or emotion, the bigger the memory. As a general rule, we only remember changes in the body and our environment that have caused some kind of an emotional response. We can't experience our world apart from the emotional response we have to it.

Feelings motivate us to action.

Without feelings it is very difficult to act. Emotions change our physical ability to move and behave. The biochemistry created when we experience emotions actually sends signals to the muscles and organs in our body that it is time to prepare to do something. There are three general categories of motivation: approach, avoid, or attack. If the emotion is positive, it will motivate us to approach and learn. If it is negative, or creates a sense of danger, we will be motivated to avoid or attack. We were created this way. Our bodies and brains were made to work together so we can learn and grow, interact with safe people, and also be safe and able to protect ourselves and the people around us.

Feelings help us communicate with others.

Did you know that we have special receptors in our brains, called mirror neurons, that help us understand what facial expressions mean in others, and then help us feel the same thing? When we see someone smile, it is natural for us to smile back. When we see someone crying, it can make us tear up as well. Our mirror neurons help create empathy. This is why we have emotions, and express them in our body language and facial expressions. We need them to communicate to others what we feel, so that we can be comforted, celebrated with, or just understood.

Research has shown that our greatest mental and emotional need, as humans, is to be validated. Validation makes us know we are real, our thoughts are real, and our feelings are real. When we express our emotions through words, facial expressions, body language, or actions, we give opportunity for others to validate our experience. We also have the opportunity to validate other people's experience and emotion when we see their emotions play out.

What happens when emotions take over?

It's all good and well when our positive emotions are in control. Our lives go along great when we feel things like joy, contentment, love, pride, or motivation. However, sometimes emotions can feel out of control, like they are in charge of our lives. They hijack us. At times emotions are all consuming, make it hard to do anything productive.

Our experience of emotion is actually just brain chemistry. That sounds a little cold, but it's true. We were created with a brain that is able to capture every piece of data that comes our way. Our brain can interpret that data at an alarming speed, even faster than a computer. Our brain decides what data is important and what is not. Then it tells us what to do with the important data. This is when chemicals and hormones are secreted into our brains to let us feel emotion, call us to action, and help us think.

The problem is that our brains don't always interpret the data exactly the way we would like. It doesn't intuitively know the past from the present. It triggers, or activates, past experiences in order to interpret current ones. Most of the time this is done without our awareness. Sometimes this becomes a problem.

When memories of negative events are triggered, our brains activate our Sympathetic and Parasympathetic nervous systems. The activation of the Sympathetic Nervous System causes us to go into a mode of fight, flight, freeze. When this activation happens, our attention is captured. We have no choice but to pay attention to our emotion. This is when we feel overwhelmed, unable to think clearly, and sometimes just shut down. I talk more about this in chapter 8.

The activation of the Parasympathetic Nervous System brings us to a state of balance. It helps calm down and come back to *normal* (whatever that is!). It is the system we want to help activate when we feel anxious and overwhelmed.

This book will talk about how essential oils can help with the process of calming the nervous system. The molecules in essential oils work perfectly with the makeup of our brain to help balance our emotions.

Let's talk about how these molecules actually work.

CHAPTER 3
AM I CRAZY, OR DO THESE OILS REALLY WORK?
ANSWERS FOR SKEPTICS & POO-POOERS

I am not a big fan of stuff I don't understand. I am always trying to figure out how things work. Essential oils are no different. When I started using essential oils it was important for me to know that this was a real thing, that there was science behind how they work in the body.

I asked my counseling team what they wanted me to write about in this book. Crystal pipes up and said, "Am I crazy, or do these oils really work?". I think we all have the same question. It seems odd that we would put lavender over our heart because we love the smell, and it calms our anxiety. We all want to know how these oils actually work in our bodies to support emotional wellness. Why are they so effective?

And what do we do with the skeptics in our lives who say that they are just placebos? My husband used to call them my "hippy oils".

There are books and books about the chemistry of essential oils. I have a book on my desk, written by David Stewart, titled *The Chemistry of Essential Oils Made Easy.* This book has 848 pages. This is just one book out of hundreds you can buy to help you understand the complex science behind essential oils. Unless you are a biochemist you may have difficulty understanding exactly what happens in our body to create the change.

I want to make this easy for everyone to understand. I want to make it short and sweet and to the point. But I am not a biochemist. I am a therapist who struggles with math and science. I had to find someone who could teach me this information in a way I could learn. I was never happier than when I found Dr. Doug Corrigan. He is a biochemist who knows all about essential oils. A great deal of my understanding about the therapeutic use of oils, and how they work in the body, comes from his teaching.

I highly recommend that you go visit his website *https://www.starfishscents.com*. He also has a book that I highly recommend, "*Innoilvation: The Science of Producing Powerful and Safe Essential Oils*". He is a fantastic teacher who is able to teach difficult concepts in a way everyone can understand.

What is an essential oil?

Essential oils are created in plants to defend it from danger, and support its health. Each essential oil consists of 12 to 300 different molecules. This is important because the balance of the molecules helps created balance in our bodies. They are small molecules that absorb into our cells easily because they dissolve into fats. Once essential oils are introduced they will be in the bloodstream within approximately two minutes. They work fast because our body was made to work with them.

When we are concerned about how essential oils work therapeutically, we only have western medicine with which to compare. Here are a few things to know:

- Essential oil molecules are around the same size as most pharmaceutical molecules.

- Essential oils can address specific problems with our physical or emotional health. They are created with many molecules that work together to balance the cell and reduce side effects.

- Pharmaceuticals can also address specific problems with our physical or emotional health. However, they have only one molecule which creates imbalance in the cellular network and can create any number of side effects.

- Over 50% of all pharmaceuticals are made from essential oil molecules. The process of separating the molecules is what can create the imbalance and produce side effects.

My response to *skeptics* and *"poo-pooers"*

There are people in my life, and I am sure yours, who have difficulty believing that essential oils can have significant therapeutic impact on our bodies and brains. Even our own experience is readily dismissed by people who believe, "It's all in your head."

When that happens I am usually okay with it. I know, for the most part, people only try things out of their comfort zone when they are desperate. I know, at some point, most people will be willing to try essential oils because they have nothing to lose and everything to gain. I know just because someone is a skeptic now, does not mean they won't be a believer later. Most of the time I am willing to let time run its course and just be available to share when they ask.

There are times when people are willing to change their minds, but they just want some more "sciencey" evidence. In this case I often will sit down with them, at a computer, and go to "Google Scholar." Over a half million articles have been published covering the impact of essential oils on wellness. There is no shortage of *real science* behind their therapeutic benefits.

Essential oils are not just some fad. They are not a bandwagon that people are on that will go away when the newness wears off. Essential oils have been used for thousands and thousands of years, and through many cultures. Some of these ancient cultures have libraries on how to use these oils for health reasons, and their effects on the body over time. Western pharmaceuticals are new to this game. They are the experiment.

In the 19th and 20th century modern day aromatherapy emerged. All over the world (Europe, Asia, Africa, etc.) doctors wrote scripts for both pharmaceuticals and essential oils. This is still a common practice today. These physicians understand that plants contain incredible medicinal qualities that help people get better. In our culture this is hard to grasp. We fall short in the area of natural medicine. The drug companies make a concerted effort to keep the public's focus on their products. However, what these companies don't want to share is that they have seen the benefit of these plants and use them in their drugs.

More and more people are testifying about the impact that essential oils have had on their health and wellness. We find books, blogs, social media posts, and hear conversations all around us describing the life changing things that happen when people start using oils. It can't be denied. Essential oils do something.

You have your own story too. I have a story. I have seen my family and friends change the way they live because of essential oils. I have seen the benefits of using them for myself. I have experienced improved emotional and physical balance. I know oils really work. That is truth.

And this is the last thing I need to say here. "Yes, Crystal... you may be crazy... but essential oils really do work!!"

ESSENTIALLY BETTER

CHAPTER 4
ALL OILS ARE NOT CREATED EQUAL

When I began researching essential oils and using them in my clinic, I wanted to make sure that I had the best oils on the market. I didn't just want them to smell nice, I wanted them to work. These were not just going to be for me. I saw the benefits that essential oils could have and I was planning on using them for my clients, and even more importantly, my family! And my family includes "the most important ones", my grandchildren! After looking into what was on the market, and doing a lot of research on the importance of consistent purity of the oils, I came to the conclusion that I would not use anything but Young Living. The reason is their *Seed to Seal* process.

Young living has a patented "Seed to Seal" process. There are 5 components: Seed, Cultivate, Distill, Test, and Seal. This is important because, as we learned in the previous chapter, essential oils have complex compounds and are made up of 20-300 different molecules. They work in our body by attaching to proteins in our cells. Because of this, it is important to know that every component (molecule) matters. The whole complex mixture of the components needs to be consistently pure in order for the oil to do what it is intended to do. Companies who want to label their products as "therapeutic grade" must meet purity standards and do so consistently. These standards must be measurable so they know that what they are selling is going to work.

Let's take a look at each one of these steps:

Seed:

When you are choosing essential oils you need to know that they start with a pure and healthy seed. This is where everything comes from. The sourcing of the seed is vital to the quality of the end product. Young Living hand chooses seeds with the highest levels of bioactive compounds (that's a good thing).

Cultivate:

Young Living predominantly owns, or partners with existing farms in order to cultivate the purest essential oils. All co-op farm practices are verified and overseen in order to match all of their proprietary standards.

When you choose an essential oil, the location and soil in which they are grown, as well as the time and method of harvesting, can produce the purest oils possible.

Some Questions to Ask About the Soil:

Do they use pesticides? Were there pesticides used on that soil in recent years? How nutritious and healthy is the soil for the specific plant they are growing? What organisms live in the soil? What is the weather like in that region of the world? Has the weather impacted the quality of the soil?

Young Living does not ever use man made pesticides, or use soil where pesticides have been used. Aftermarket testing has been conducted on a number of essential oil brands where pesticides were present in the oil. This is rather startling. The purity and quality of the soil is so important.

Some Questions to Ask About Harvesting Practices:

What time of year do you harvest your plants? What time of month? Time of day? What part of the plant do your oils come from? What equipment do you use to harvest? How do you make decisions about your harvesting practices?

Did you know that the time of year matters in harvesting? The quality and strength of some oils can be affected by harvesting at the wrong time of month, while others are impacted even by the time of day. For oils to be consistently effective a company needs to harvest the plants at the peak time.

It is important that you choose a company who is informed about the science of harvesting practices, and who is in control of this process for their plants. Most companies purchase plants after they are harvested. They have had no control over these practices. Young Living monitors all of their harvesting practices and, by doing so, keeps consistency in the quality of their oils.

Because of the control they have over the farms where their plants are grown, Young Living is also able to choose, and confirm the part of the plant from which their oils are extracted.

Distill:

Young Living always distills their own oils from the plant. They continue to be on the cutting-edge of innovation when it comes to distilling oil.

Some Questions to Ask About Distillation Practices:

What equipment do you use to distill? What different kinds of distillation processes do you use? How long do you distill each oil? At what temperature and pressure? Is your equipment steel or are there any plastic parts?

Young Living controls the whole process of distillation and uses no plastic parts on their machinery. Plasticides have been found in oils from other companies because of the distillation process they use (yuck!!).

Young Living uses both cold press and steam processes to extract oils. For years they have studied and perfected the length of time, temperature, and pressure they use to distill oils so that it is the purest, and most consistent oil on the planet. All of these processes are patented and are proprietary to the company.

Test:

Young Living tests more than any other oil company in the world. Each essential oil is tested in their own state of the art lab. They also use two different independent, accredited labs to test their oils with different methods.
Young Living has the highest standards in the industry for the quality of oils that they will sell to their customers. I like that!

Seal:

Young Living uses clean rooms to bottle their oils. This insures the purity of the oils we buy. They bottle all of their essential oils in UV-protective amber glass so that the oils can maintain their potency and quality. The pure oils will never go bad over time.

These aren't just oils to make your house smell like a spa, these are oils used for therapeutic interventions. We want them to be pure, like we want our medications to be pure. Don't settle for poor quality. You have chosen to use oils for the good things that they can do for your body. You are worth the best!

ESSENTIALLY BETTER

CHAPTER 5
START WITH THE MUST HAVE LIST
~DR. BRUTON'S EMOTIONAL OIL EMERGENCY KIT~

Choosing where to start can be overwhelming. Many people, including myself, get a Young Living Premium Starter Kit (PSK) and then don't know what to do with it. It feels like there is so much to learn…and so much to buy.

The truth is that there is a very long list of oils that work for emotional balance and wellbeing. Just like medications, each person may respond better or worse to specific oils. This is why I have suggested several oils for each issue.

A friend of mine told me she wished I would have a "must have list" of 5 oils. Sorry Rachel, I couldn't do it. BUT I decided I could do a *Top 5 Single Oils* and a *Top 5 Oil Blends.* These are in addition to the oils that are available in the PSK.

Here are my Emotional Oil Emergency Kits. My hope is this will give you a place to start.

Single Oils:	**Blends:**
Bergamot	Peace & Calming
Ylang Ylang	Trauma Life
Vetiver	Hope
Cedarwood	Envision
Tangerine	Gathering

NOTE: Young Living has three kits that are wonderful. I love them. I have all of them!! As you begin to feel more comfortable using these oils, I would suggest investing in one or more of these kits.

- The Feelings Kit
- The Freedom Sleep Kit
- The Freedom Release Kit

I will talk about these kits at the end of this chapter.

Dr. Bruton's Emergency Kit #1: Single Oils

Bergamot: Bergamot is a very well rounded oil. Its key constituents are readily used by the amygdala and hippocampus (the emotion center of the brain). It has been traditionally used for calming and providing hormonal support. It is used for reducing stress and increasing appetite. It helps fight agitation, depression, anxiety, and nervous tension. Jean Valnet, MD, recommends it as an antidepressant, and to regulate appetite (Young, 2003).

This oil is an overall great oil to use any time you need to regulate emotions or are having difficulty tolerating distress.

How to use Bergamot:

- *Diffuse*: Diffuse alone or with other oils. 2-3 times a day or directly from your hands for 2-3 minutes.
- *Topically*: neck, wrists, over the heart, or on the top of the head.

Ylang Ylang: I love the smell of *Ylang Ylang*. It is a happy smell to me! This oil is known to help balance blood pressure and regulate your heartbeat. It helps bring more spiritual awareness and promotes positive thinking. It helps calm rapid breathing, balance equilibrium, and ease frustration. It is indicated for anxiety, depression, mental fatigue, and insomnia.

Another fun thing to note is that *Ylang Ylang* also helps increase libido. In the Philippines and Indonesia, the Ylang Ylang flowers were used to cover the beds of newlywed couples on their wedding night (Young, 2003).

I use this oil often. It seems to work well for me when I need to relax or calm down. It is a good overall body regulator.

How to use Ylang Ylang:

- *Diffuse*: Diffuse alone or with other oils. 2-3 times a day or directly from your hands for 2-3 minutes.
- *Topically*: Use 2-3 drops on the neck, wrists, over the heart, down the spine, or on the top of the head.

Vetiver: This is my go-to oil for focus. It is used in conjunction with Cedarwood to help you when you are scattered, distracted, and anxious. It is a very thick oil (*trick:* I take the inside lid off the bottle and use a dropper because I don't have enough patience to wait for it to come out). Vetiver is very grounding. It settles the nervous system, and stimulates the circulatory system. It has been used to decrease anxiety and depression (Young, 2003).

This is a good oil to use when you need to increase mindfulness and focus.

How to use Vetiver:
- *Diffuse*: I prefer to inhale this directly from the hands (mixed with Cedarwood) for 2-3 minutes. Do this 3-4 times a day for several days. This will help balance your system so you won't need to do it as often.
- *Topically*: This is the best way to use this oil. Use 2-3 drops on the neck, wrists, over the heart, down the spine, or on the top of the head.

Cedarwood: This oil actually stimulates the limbic region of the brain. This is the emotion center of our brains. Cedarwood is an excellent oil for releasing nervous tension, and regulating emotion. It also helps balance our ability to think and feel at the same time. Cedarwood helps our bodies release melatonin so that our sleep is much deeper.

Cedarwood, combined with vetiver or bergamot, is my go to combo for grounding and focus.

How to use Cedarwood:
- *Diffuse*: This can be combined with other oils in a diffuser (I love the smell of Cedarwood & Joy) Diffuse several times a day, or all night with Peace & Calming for a great night's sleep. You can also inhale this directly from the hands (mixed with vetiver) for 2-3 minutes.
- *Topically*: This is a very effective way to use this oil. Use 2-3 drops on the neck, wrists, over the heart, down the spine, top of head, or bottom of the feet.

Tangerine: I know I keep saying this, but I love this oil! It is really one of my top 3 oils I like to smell. It lifts my spirits every time I use it. I often have it on a diffuser bracelet with Peppermint (and just FYI, Peppermint is in your starter kit so I didn't include it on my emergency kit... but it would have been there if you didn't already have it!!).

Tangerine makes you nothing but happy. It helps decrease anxiety and nervousness. Tangerine has also been used to help with insomnia. My guess is that it helps with sleep because you are so much happier and less anxious. (Have I said I really like this oil???)

(Just a side note: Tangerine has been known to help with stretch marks and fluid retention too. That can only be a good thing!)

If you come to my house or office you will undoubtedly find at least one diffuser going filled with tangerine and peppermint. This is my pick-me-up oil combo that I need almost every day.

How to use Tangerine:
- *Diffuse*: Diffuse this oil all day long. I have said I like it with Peppermint, but I also love it with Stress Away. You can also inhale this directly from the hands (mixed with whatever you like) for 2-3 minutes.
- *Topically*: This is a very effective way to use this oil. Use 2-3 drops on the neck, wrists, over the heart, down the spine, top of head, or bottom of the feet.
- *Orally*: Put 1-2 drops in your water! It makes it so fresh and good.

Dr. Bruton's Emergency Kit #2: Blends

Peace & Calming: I can't say enough about *Peace & Calming*. Mostly because it puts all three of my grandsons to sleep in minutes. I do have to say that a lot of people don't have this same experience and have difficulty sleeping with this oil. However, for my family it works wonders. It also seems to calm my soul. You know the part of you that can feel unsettled even when you seem calm? That's the part of me that gets to rest when I use this oil.

Among other things, it is used for comfort, patience, meditation, and letting go of anxiety.

Here are the oils that are in *Peace & Calming*: Ylang Ylang, Orange, Tangerine, Patchouli, and Blue Tansy.

How to use Peace & Calming:
- *Diffuse*: Diffuse this oil all day long. I love to use it with *Citrus Fresh* or *Peppermint.* I encourage you to experiment and see what combinations you can find. My husband and I diffuse *Peace & Calming* and *Trauma Life* every night.
- *Topically*: This is a very effective way to use this oil. Use 2-3 drops on the neck, wrists, over the heart, down the spine, top of head, or bottom of the feet.
- *In a Bath*: Add 4-5 drops to 1 cup Epsom salts and put it in your bath at night. This is so relaxing. I love it!

Trauma Life: Trauma Life has become a go-to oil for me both professionally and personally. It is a blend that has a strong and beautiful fragrance. It helps you to mentally relax and let go of traumatic experiences and their memories. It is also a good oil to use while in counseling. This combination of oils can help in unlocking traumatic experiences. At the same time, it can also bring a sense of peace and joy to life. This is a coveted combination.

Here are the oils that are in *Trauma Life*: Sandalwood, Helichrysum, Rose, Frankincense, Valerian, Black Spruce, Davana, Lavender, Geranium, and Lime.

How to use Trauma Life:
- *Diffuse*: Diffuse this oil in times of high stress. If you are having intrusive thoughts about past trauma, this should be the first oil

you reach for. I love to use it with *Peppermint.* Many people use this oil with *Frankincense* for a calming effect. This is one of the oils that my husband and I diffuse every night. We combine it with *Peace & Calming.* It is so helpful.

- *Topically*: This is a very effective way to use this oil. Use 2-3 drops on the neck, wrists, over the heart, down the spine, top of head, or bottom of the feet.

Hope: Hope is the first oil I bought for my own emotional support. This is one of my top 2 favorite oils. *Hope & Envision* are the oils that I use every day for my own emotional wellness and balance. As I am writing this description I am struggling to come up with words that describe what this oil blend does for me. I realize that the name says it all. It gives, or activates *Hope*. When you breathe it in, this blend of oils gives you a feeling of going forward with strength. It gives a sense of grounding. At times when I feel hopeless, this oil blend has been a game changer.

Here are the oils that are in *Hope:* Sweet Almond, Melissa, Juniper, Myrrh, and Black Spruce

How to use Hope:
- *Diffuse*: I think the best way to use this oil is to inhale it directly from your hands for 2-3 minutes. I use this with *Envision* each day. The more often you use this blend, the more effective it will be in maintaining your mood. You can also put *Hope* in a diffuser. Combine it with other oils to create a happy space.

- *Topically*: Use 2-3 drops on the outer edge of the ears. It can also be placed over the heart, chest, or down your spine. I use this oil in combination with *Envision* as a perfume!

Envision: *Envision* is the next oil in my top 2 all-time favorite oils. I use it daily with *Hope.* This is a blend of oils that was designed to awaken the part of your brain that sets goals, and dreams about the future. It helps you let go of fears and move forward. If you feel stuck in life this is the oil for you. It stimulates creativity and helps you have renewed faith. (Have I said that I love this oil???)

Here are the oils that are in *Envision*: Spruce, Lavender, Rose, Orange, Geranium, and Sage

How to use Envision:

- *Diffuse*: Just like with *Hope,* I think the best way to use this oil is to inhale it directly from your hands for 2-3 minutes. I use this with *Hope* each day. The more often you use this blend, the more effective it will be in maintaining your mood. You can also put *Envision* in a diffuser. This is especially good when you are in a meeting with others, planning future events, or dreaming about possibilities.

- *Topically*: Use 2-3 drops on the outer edge of the ears or forehead. It can also be placed over the heart, chest, or bottom of the feet. I use this oil in combination with *Hope* as a perfume!

Gathering: When I first saw the name of this oil I was curious about what it was intended to do. As I read more about it I loved the name. This blend of oils was made to help us gather our inner strength, both spiritual and emotional strength. It combines two different oils that were used by Moses for incense, galbanum and frankincense. When our brains are able to weed through the chaotic energy around us every day, we can focus better and achieve greater things.

This is also a great oil to use to help stop arguing or conflict in your home. Put this blend on kiddos when they are unsettled or angry with each other. It can help stop the bickering that drives you crazy. (By the way... this doesn't just work with kiddos, it works with your partners too!)

Here are the oils that are in *Gathering*: Lavender, Geranium, Galbanum, Frankincense, Royal Hawaiian Sandalwood, Ylang Ylang, Black Spruce, Cinnamon, and Rose

How to use *Gathering*:

- *Diffuse*: You can also put *Gathering* in a diffuser with other oils like *Frankincense.* This is a great way to help you make a creative atmosphere.

- *Topically*: Use 2-3 drops on the outer edge of the ears or forehead. It can also be placed over the heart, chest, or bottom of the feet. This blend is often used on the spine. I use this oil, in combination with *Harmony,* to help stop conflicts in my home and in my office.

Those are my top emotional wellness picks. I wanted to give you a place to start when choosing essential oils for yourself or loved ones.

Another option is to start with the kits developed by Young Living to specifically address emotional needs. They have three kits. I hope you give them a try over time.

Young Living's Feelings Kit:

This is a kit that was designed by Young Living to promote emotional wellness and self-renewal.

Please Note: At times Young Living changes the oils that are in the kit. Here is what is in the kit at the time this book was published.

Oil Blends in the Feelings Kit: Valor, Harmony, Forgiveness, Present Time, Release, Inner Child

Young Living's Freedom Sleep Kit:

This kit was created to work with the energy flow throughout the body. It helps improve your ability to relax and let go of your racing thoughts. This kit has been used with war veterans with wonderful results.

Oil Blends in the Freedom Sleep Kit: Freedom, AromaSleep, Inner Harmony, and Valor

Young Living's Freedom Release Kit:

This kit was developed by Dr. Gary Young specifically for war Veterans. It has shown some fabulous results. This combination of oils helps bring a sense of balance and harmony, while allowing for the release of anger.

Oil Blends in the Freedom Release Kit: Freedom, Divine Release, Joy, Transformation, and T.R. Care

Part 2

Essential Oils for People with Feelings

INTRO TO PART 2
ESSENTIAL OILS FOR PEOPLE WITH FEELINGS

In this section I will be talking about 10 different mental health issues which, in my experience, are among the most common reasons people seek counseling. These are also the things that make our lives hard and cause us a lot of distress. The problem is that even though someone might be given a diagnosis by a mental health professional or a physician, it is not the diagnosis that makes them miserable... it is the way in which this diagnosis plays out in their life. This is where essential oils can help.

In the next several chapters I will be discussing 10 different mental health issues and what symptoms are associated with them. These specific symptoms come both from the Diagnostic & Statistical Manual (DSM-5) and my clinical experience. At times the language has been changed to clarify, in everyday terms, what actually is happening. Please hear me... this is important. **I am in no way asserting that essential oils can cure mental health disorders.** For that matter, neither can pharmaceuticals. My intention is to connect symptoms that come with specific diagnoses, with a list of oils that could support wellness in these areas.

In this section, I will outline some of the symptoms that can occur within each mental health issue. Then I will be discussing different essential oils that could support your body while moving toward wellness. Each person is uniquely made. This means that each person will experience a different combination of emotional and behavioral symptoms. A therapist or physician can give two people the same diagnosis, though their symptoms may be very different. For example, there are over 300 combinations of symptoms that are possible to be diagnosed with Borderline Personality Disorder. There only needs to be 5 of the 12 criteria met in order to diagnose. So not every person with a specific disorder has the same symptoms. Because of this, not everyone should use the same oils… or the same pharmaceuticals. It is important to know this!

After the list of symptoms, I will be talking about interventions that have been helpful when working with people with these issues. I am including this because in the vast majority of cases, the combination of therapy, essential oils, and/or pharmaceuticals leads to the best outcomes. Please always talk to your physician and therapist about what you are using and what you would like to use to help support your emotional wellness.

CHAPTER 6
ADJUSTING TO A NEW NORMAL

Everyone... and I mean EVERYONE... who has lived life for a while has had to learn to adjust to a "new normal." But, there are times when this adjustment throws us off our game and into a tailspin of emotions and poor behavior. It is what happens when you have an event in your life that takes you by surprise, and you find it difficult to handle (i.e.: divorce, moving, changing jobs, losing a job, or even death of a loved one). These things that happen to us are called **stressors**. Because of these stressors, people can find themselves struggling to find emotional balance, and have difficulty behaving the way they would normally behave.

Symptoms and Impact:

People who struggle with adjusting to hard events could have any or all of these experiences...

- Developing feelings or actions that are outside of what is normal for you within 3 months of the stressor

- The emotions you feel are out of proportion for the event that happened.
- These emotions and actions are causing problems in several places in your life (i.e.: work, home, friendships, school)
- The way it looks can be different for everyone. You can experience any of the following:
  - Extreme sadness
  - Tearfulness
  - Hopelessness
  - Worry
  - Nervousness
  - Fear
  - Separation Anxiety
  - Acting or behaving outside of your norm
  - Having reactions that are not healthy for your circumstances

A Note on Grief: When we have someone close to us die, our world can feel like it has fallen apart. We feel like everything is moving faster than we are able to handle. No matter what the circumstances surrounding the death of someone in our life, it is one of the most difficult things for our psyches to manage. We were not created to accept death right away; we have to grieve. It is a process, one that is ugly, messy, hard, and painful. Although grief is not a "mental health disorder" it most certainly can make us unsteady on our emotional feet. All of the following discussion can be applied to the grieving process. We need to take care of ourselves throughout our time in grief. Pay attention to what you need. Nurture your heart, soul, body, and mind.

Common Treatments:

Counseling: As a therapist, most of the people I see are working through some significant stressor that has happened to them. They want help working through the feelings and actions that have taken them by surprise. They need skills to learn to cope with a "new normal" in their life.

This is a normal experience for many of us. However when things happen in life that make it hard for us to cope, our brains sometimes feel like there is a heavy fog over us. It makes it difficult to think clearly, make decisions, or be effective in our daily life. Talking with someone outside of friends or family (talk therapy) can be very helpful in sorting out the feelings and actions that seem unclear in our heads. Good counselors have the ability to reflect what you are saying, and to clarify the cloudy and muddled experience going on in your head. Good counselors also can help give you skills that will make it easier to focus, reason, and regulate your emotions and actions more effectively. Finding a good therapist is one of the best things you can do for yourself, and the people you love, when you find yourself trying to adjust to a "new normal."

If your counselor doesn't use essential oils during your sessions, let them know that incorporating *essential oils* in your counseling sessions can increase the effectiveness of your time together.

Some skills that may help while adjusting to a "new normal":

Mindfulness: focus, observing your surroundings nonjudgmentally, being "in the moment"

Breathing Exercises: square breathing (see *All the Things*)

Personal Yoga Practice

Emotional Regulation Skills
- Sleep
- Exercise
- Do something you are good at… or learn something new
- Act opposite to your emotion (i.e., if you are sad, watch a comedy or listen to a fun song)

Distress Tolerance Skills
- Self-sooth with your five senses: do something for each sense (taste, smell, sight, hearing, touch) that is calming and comforting.
- Distracting
- Radical Acceptance

Pharmaceuticals: There are no pharmaceuticals that are created for this specific issue. Sometimes physicians will prescribe antidepressants or anti-anxiety medications for symptom relief. However, these medications were not created for this issue.

Essential Oils for Adjusting to a *New Normal*:

Essential oils are highly effective for this issue. The brain is made to work in tandem with essential oils to effectively help regulate emotions and thoughts, and in turn, our behavior. Most of the time we are not dealing with adjusting to a new normal for more than a few months at a time. Essential oils are a strong addition to any wellness plan you are making as you move through hard transitions.

Here is a list of the symptoms we talked about earlier, and some essential oils that research has shown to help support emotional wellness in these areas. This is by no means an exhaustive list. These are my favorites and what I have seen be the most effective in my work with clients. (* oil blends)

Extreme Sadness:
- Bergamot
- Joy*
- Peppermint
- Clary Sage
- Ylang Ylang
- Grapefruit

Tearfulness:
- Acceptance*
- Sandalwood
- Clary Sage
- Patchouli
- Valor*
- Ylang Ylang
- Melissa
- Rose

Hopelessness:
- Hope*
- Geranium
- Envision*
- Roman Chamomile
- Sandalwood
- Orange

Worry & Nervousness:
- Acceptance*
- Lavender
- Stress Away*
- Joy*
- Bergamot
- Copaiba

Fear:
- Valor*
- Vetiver
- Cedarwood
- Copaiba
- Peppermint
- Envision*
- Grapefruit
- Bergamot

Separation Anxiety:
- Peace & Calming*
- Melissa
- Lavender
- Cedarwood
- Bergamot
- Orange
- Lemon
- Acceptance*

Acting or behaving outside of your norm and in unhealthy ways:
- Vetiver
- Clarity
- Cedarwood
- Forgiveness*
- Gratitude*
- Focus*

Grief
- Neroli
- Rose
- Lavender
- Melissa
- Roman Chamomile
- Vetiver
- Patchouli
- Frankincense

Dr. B's Top 3 oils for *Adjusting to a New Normal:*

- Hope*
- Acceptance*
- Envision*

How do I use these oils?:

In the chapter on how essential oils work I talked about different ways to use oils. All three ways of using oils can be effective when dealing with these emotions. We have seen the greatest impact when the oils are *diffused or inhaled* from your hand. This is because the emotion center of the brain is so close to the olfactory bulb... the oil molecules go directly to the place they are needed. All of these oils can be used in diffusers. They can also be put in your hand (a drop or two of a couple of your favorites) and breath in for 2-3 minutes. This is a good time to do the square breathing exercise I talked about earlier.

All of these oils can also be put on your body and absorbed into the skin. Here is a list of effective places to put them for these specific issues:

- Over your heart
- Back of your neck
- Earlobe
- Wrist
- Bottom of the feet

Ingesting some of the oils from Young Living's *vitality* line would also be helpful if you wanted to try them. Peppermint, lemon, orange, or grapefruit are some of my favorites.

For Counselors & Helpers:

I want to encourage you to use these oils in session with clients who have been stuck in the same place for a few weeks/months. Here are some suggestions for integrating oils into a counseling session... try one or all of them:

- Ask if you can diffuse during session.

- Ask if they would be willing to put a few drops of oils on the palms of their hands and breathe in the aroma.
- Do a breathing exercise at the beginning of session with oils.
- Pay attention to the changes.
- Ask your client "what are you noticing in..."
  - Your body
  - Your mood

Most of all, you need to pay attention to differences you see in their body posture and facial expressions. Point out the changes.

I suggest you re-apply oils half way through the session. Let them take a minute to breathe in the oils again. Make sure to keep the diffuser running throughout the session.

Notes & Oils List

_____

_____

_____

_____

_____

_____

_____

CHAPTER 7
SADNESS… DEEP, DEEP SADNESS

There are times in life that the word "sadness" isn't strong enough to describe what you are feeling. It can be brought on by an event like we talked about in the previous chapter, or sometimes it just happens. Our brains were made to perfectly balance our bodies and moods. We have chemicals and hormones in our brain which, when balanced, create happiness, the ability to cope, and an overall sense of wellbeing. When, for whatever reason, our brain chemistry gets out of balance, our mood and body change. This can happen because of hard circumstances, physical illness, change of seasons, or just change in our hormones from aging. *Deep, Deep Sadness* creates all kinds of issues in our lives. It impacts our ability to function in our families, at work, with friends, and often is personally shaming.

Symptoms and Impact:

More than perhaps any other mental health issue, this issue looks different in everyone. There are some symptoms that are common to the experience, but the combination of symptoms will vary with each individual.

Here is a list of things that might be happening if you are in a place of *Deep, Deep Sadness:*

- Sad or numb feeling most of the day, nearly every day.
- No interest in doing things that used to be fun or exciting.
- Difficulty finding pleasure from things, people, or events that used to bring joy.
- Eating a lot... more than normal
- Eating very little with no appetite.
- Difficulty sleeping
- Crying for no specific reason
- Sleeping all the time: difficulty getting out of bed, and rarely feel rested.
- Slow moving...
  May include speaking slower or moving slower than normal.
- No energy; Fatigue. May include feeling pain in the body.
- Feeling worthless and guilty
- Feelings of hopelessness
- Difficulty concentrating or decision making
- Impaired memory
- Sometimes there can be recurring and pervasive thoughts about death or dying.

A Note on Suicide & Suicidal Thoughts: When people find themselves in this deep place of sadness it is easy, and normal, to start entertaining thoughts like "everyone would be better off without me", or "I feel so much pain, I can't handle this anymore." This is a dangerous place to be and needs to be taken seriously. There is help… and hope. Call your local crisis line, your physician, or your therapist. Call a friend, family member, or your neighbor. Take a deep breath and let someone know what you're are feeling and thinking. What feels overwhelming and permanent will pass, and it will get better. I promise.

https://suicidepreventionlifeline.org

Common Treatments:

Counseling: When people are experiencing these symptoms it is often difficult to find the energy to go anywhere, let alone to a therapist. This is true especially if you don't have a relationship with a counselor already. Finding a good counselor to walk with you through these times can be life-changing.

When in counseling the therapist can give you skills to manage some of the symptoms. The counselors also can create a safe space to express all of the thoughts and feelings inside you that may become difficult for your family and friends to hear. They are often ablc to validate your experience, and just listen much better because they are not connected to you in any other place in life. Expressing the feelings out loud can be transformative.

If there is a specific event that triggered this sadness, good counselors can help you process the event in a way that is both healthy and holistic.

Remember that incorporating *essential oils* in your counseling sessions can increase the effectiveness of your time together.

Some skills that may help when in a deep sadness:

Mindfulness: Being "In the Moment"
- *What is happening right now*? Are you thinking about the past? The future? Let go of those things and notice what is happening in the "here and now". What is happening in your body? What do you feel that is comfortable? Focus on the NOW.

Breathing Exercises: (See the *All The Stuff* section at the end of the book.)
- Square Breathing
- Bilateral nostril breathing

Personal Yoga Practice: Study after study has shown that having a regular yoga practice is an effective way to enhance mood. A lifted mood is only one of many benefits of yoga

Emotional Regulation Skills
- Create good sleep hygiene: Sleep is very important for this specific issue of deep sadness. Sleep is thrown off when our brains are sad. It becomes a vicious cycle. (See the "Sleep Hygiene Protocol" in *All The Stuff* section at the end of the book)
- Exercise: I hate exercise... really!! But for this issue it is vital that you move... just move. It will go against everything in you to

move, but do it anyway. It is so important. Get up and MOVE!

- Do something you are good at or learn something new.
- Act opposite to your emotion: our emotions are like little stray cats. They need to be fed to grow and stay around. They will do everything they can to get fed, but remember: DON'T FEED THE WILD ANIMALS! Feed them when they are good and you want to have them around. But don't feed them if you want them to leave. Do something opposite. It won't feel right, but do it anyway. Act "as if" you are happy and feeling joy. Act "as if" you have energy. Act "as if" you like being around people. Our brains want us to *feel our way into a better way of acting…* but the truth is that we often have to *act our way into a better way of feeling.*

Distress Tolerance Skills

- Self-sooth with your five senses: do something for each sense (taste, smell, sight, hearing, touch) that is calming and comforting.
- Distracting: don't sit and think about all of the sad, horrible things that have happened and could happen. Distract yourself with something else, anything else: Watch TV, play loud music, call a friend, go for a walk. Get your mind off the things that make you sad.

Talk to People Around You, and Listen to Their Stories.

- Understanding and empathizing with others is one of the best ways to regulate mood.
- Find positive people and mimic their facial expressions: when we smile our brain chemistry changes. Yes! Our mood changes our facial expressions, but our facial expressions can change our mood too. Try it and see what happens.

Pharmaceuticals: When people have deep, deep sadness for a significant period of time (more than 1 month) it is important for them to go see a physician or a psychiatric nurse practitioner.

There are so many good pharmaceuticals that can help regulate your mood. Many times an antidepressant or a mood stabilizer will be prescribed. However, they are not all the same. If one does not work, you can ask to try another one.

When you need medication it is very important that you take it as prescribed and don't go off of it without the help of your prescriber. If you have found a medication that has helped you, but you have side effects that are concerning to you, it is a good time to try adding essential oils. The complex molecules in essential oils help balance the cellular network that has been disrupted by pharmaceuticals.

Essential Oils for Deep, Deep Sadness:

Feelings of Extreme Sadness.
- Hope
- Neroli
- Joy*
- St. John's Wort
- Lavender
- Lemon

Feeling Numb
- Peppermint
- Joy*
- Envision*
- Vetiver
- Lavender
- Bergamot

Lack of Interest
- Hope*
- Envision*
- Valor*
- Purification*
- Motivation*
- Peppermint

Lack of Ability to find Pleasure
- Cedarwood
- Vetiver
- Joy*
- Motivation*
- Peppermint
- Tangerine

Over Eating
- Grapefruit
- Lime
- Peppermint
- Lemon
- Copaiba
- Lavender

No Appetite
- Bergamot
- Taragon
- Cedarwood
- Fennel
- Copaiba
- Nutmeg

Difficulty Sleeping
- Bergamot
- Vetiver
- Ylang Ylang
- Cedarwood
- Lavender
- Sleep Essence*

Sleeping all the time: difficulty getting out of bed, rarely feel rested.
- Peppermint
- Tangerine
- En-R Gee*
- Purification*
- Motivation*
- Jasmine

Unprovoked Crying Episodes
- Rose
- Neroli
- Sandalwood
- Roman Chamomile
- Ylang Ylang
- White Angelica

Slow Movements & Speech
- Peppermint
- Grapefruit
- Eucalyptus
- Tangerine
- En-R-Gee*
- Motivation*

Lack of Energy~ Fatigue
- Grapefruit
- Helichrysum
- Clary Sage
- Joy*
- Motivation*
- En-R-Gee*

Feelings of Worthlessness & Guilt
- Valor*
- Forgiveness*
- Hope*
- Gratitude*
- Orange
- Tangerine

Feelings of Hopelessness
- Hope*
- Envision*
- Peace & Calming*
- Joy*
- Valor*
- Ylang-Ylang

Difficulty Concentrating or Making Decisions
- Basil
- Vetiver
- Peppermint
- Clarity*
- Cardamom
- En-R-Gee*

Impaired Memory
- Clarity*
- Mind Wise*
- Rose
- Rosemary
- Vetiver
- Common Sense*

Thoughts of Death & Dying
- Acceptance*
- Ylang Ylang
- Vetiver
- Rose
- Melissa
- Tangerine

Dr. B's top 3 oils for Deep, Deep Sadness:

- Bergamot
- En-R-Gee*
- Hope*

How do I use these oils?:

There are a lot of oils listed in this section. The fact is that most essential oils help with uplifting our mood. I am in no way suggesting you get all of them. I just want you to try a few. See what works best for you. These oils work well blended. I would suggest diffusing two or three that you think would be good together and see if it is helpful. The best way to get oils to your brain where you need It is to use your hands as a diffuser and inhale for 2-3 minutes. Look at the rollerball recipes in the *All The Stuff* section at the back of the book. There are several recipes there that would work for this issue. Be creative. Try new things. Experiment. Ask people you know what they are using for sadness.

Here are the best places to put oils on your body for *Deep, Deep Sadness:*

- Feet
- Head (all over it!!)
- Heart
- Wrist

For Counselors & Helpers:

I know when I have a lot of sad clients at one time it can start to rub off on me. How about you?? We need to make sure we are taking care of ourselves as helpers. Start your sessions by putting *Peppermint* on your own wrists.

Put a drop or two of *Joy* over your heart or on your forehead. This is a technique that has helped me focus and stay present and in my own emotion instead of my client's emotion.

Start by introducing essential oils with a diffuser. Try some blends. Perhaps have some rollerballs available for clients to try. And as always, use them in breathing exercises. Notice what happens!

Notes & Oils List

_____

_____

_____

_____

_____

_____

CHAPTER 8
FEELING SUPER ANXIOUS

Anxiety is one of the worst feelings anyone can ever have! I hate it, and I know I am not the only one who feels this way. It can be all consuming. It takes over your mind, body, and soul. It's like you are taken hostage by the thoughts that keep racing through your head. It can feel so out of your control… like it's just happening to you and you don't know how to stop it. Your heart beats fast, your breath becomes shallow, your ability to interact with others becomes very limited. It's awful.

The truth is when anxiety hits, you *have* been hijacked. We have been created with a brain that is extremely vigilant about noticing where there might be danger. When our brain perceives danger around us, it signals our body to release adrenaline so that we can protect ourselves by either fighting, fleeing, or freezing. Our blood is sent to our extremities so we can run away or fight. It takes oxygen and blood from our organs and brain to protect us if we get injured. Our bodies go into a survival mode and focuses our attention on only the danger so we stay alert to it and can be safe. This is very helpful when you are in a place of physical danger, it can save your life. Once the danger is over and you have fled the scene, or fought your way out, the adrenaline has been used up and things can go back to normal. We are beautifully and wonderfully made.

The problem is that our brains don't know the difference between physical danger and emotional danger. So when our brains perceive danger, even though it is emotional, our body goes into action. Adrenaline is released into our blood system and we begin the process of figuring out if we should fight, flee, or freeze. Our heart starts racing because of the adrenaline, our breath becomes shallow, our blood goes to our extremities making us feel sick to our stomachs. We can feel light headed, struggle to think clearly, and sometimes have chest pains. Our focus is put entirely on the "danger" at hand. We can't stop thinking about the problem. It consumes us. And, unlike when we are in physical danger, we don't use up the adrenaline in our systems so it just keeps going... and going.

Everyone feels anxious sometimes. It can have some really good outcomes for us when we feel anxiety. It motivates us to do something and focuses our attention. It warns us of danger that may be there. We can have anxiety over good things like the birth of a child, or a new job. It can also happen when hard circumstances come into our lives. Either way it is a normal experience of being human. However, when this is an experience that continually happens to you, or you find yourself unable to function, this is when it becomes a problem.

When I asked people to describe their anxiety in a few words this was the response:

- panic
- breathless
- motivation
- nervous
- flustered
- debilitating
- crippling
- nagging
- all-consuming
- joy-stealing
- heavy
- hopeless
- judgmental
- scared
- demanding
- distracting
- informative
- fearful
- violating
- intrusive
- dread
- nausea
- weariness
- inaction
- rumination
- worry
- lack of control
- sleepless
- need to be alone

Symptoms and Impact:

Here is a list of symptoms that happen when you are continually *Feeling Super Anxious*

- Excessive worry (happens more days than not)
- Unable to control racing thoughts and worry
- Restlessness, feeling keyed up
- Irritable
- Paranoid
- Fear of dying
- Bodily tension (e.g. chest, neck, back, buttocks)
- Can't go to sleep

- Can't stay asleep
- Lack of concentration
- Racing Heartbeat
- Sweating
- Frequent urination or diarrhea
- Shallow Breathing or unable to catch your breath

Common Treatments:

Counseling*:* Talk therapy is one of the most effective ways to find resolution when you are continually feeling super anxious. It is important to find a good counselor who can help you process out loud what is happening in your head. One of the main troubles with anxiety is the racing thoughts that go around and around in your brain. Soon those thoughts become toxic when they have not been said out loud. They seem perfectly reasonable when they are in your head, but when you say them out loud they often lose their power. Good counselors can help by validating your experience, as well as letting you come to some resolutions for yourself. They can teach skills on how to reduce anxiety with both body and brain exercises. Incorporating essential oils in your counseling sessions can increase the effectiveness of your time together.

Some skills that may help when you feel anxious:

Mindfulness Exercises: Being able to focus on the *here and now* will help reduce the worry about tomorrow. Be aware of what is around you. Find details in little (i.e. count the shades of blue).

Focus on relaxing your pelvic floor. Your sympathetic nervous system cannot be activated when your pelvic floor is relaxed.

Breathing Exercises: Belly breathing is very good for activating the parasympathetic nervous system. Look up some different breathing exercises online. Pinterest is a great place to find exercises like this.

Yoga: Yoga can sometimes feel like torture when you are anxious, but it is exactly what you need. You need your body to move, be submissive to your brain, and learn to relax. Find a good place to do yoga!! It's important!

Progressive Muscle Relaxation: (see *All The Things* at the end of the book)

Challenging Your Own Unhelpful Thoughts: Remember, thoughts are just thoughts. They are not truth. Think about them rationally, letting go of the emotion behind them. Are they true? Change what needs to be changed and focus on facts! Google "thinking errors that trigger anxiety".

Pharmaceuticals: There are several different kinds of pharmaceuticals that are effective in reducing anxiety. The problem is that they rarely help to prevent anxiety attacks, only reduce the severity when they happen. These kinds of medications can also be extremely addictive. There are a number of side effects to medications for anxiety. However, if you need them they are very helpful. Ask your prescriber about options.

Talk to them about side effects. And, as always, use them the way they are prescribed, while supporting them with essential oils.

Essential Oils for feeling super anxious:

Excessive worry (happens more days then not)
- Peace & Calming*
- Bergamot
- Neroli
- Lavender
- Melissa
- Cedarwood

Unable to control racing thoughts and worry
- Gathering*
- Frankincense
- Vetiver
- Lavender
- Ylang Ylang
- Cedarwood

Restlessness, feeling keyed up
- Gathering*
- Grounding*
- Peace & Calming*
- Sandalwood
- Ylang Ylang
- White Angelica

Irritable
- Rose
- Cypress
- Stress Away*
- Clary Sage
- Frankincense
- Grounding*

Paranoid
- Cedarwood
- Cypress
- Peace & Calming*
- Lemongrass
- Basil
- Bergamot

Fear of dying
- Joy*
- Neroli
- Peace & Calming*
- Valor*
- Grounding*
- Gathering*

Bodily tension (e.g. chest, neck, back, buttocks)
- Stress Away*
- M-Grain*
- Aroma Siez*
- PanAway*
- Copaiba
- Wintergreen

Can't go to sleep/ Can't stay asleep
- Lavender
- Trauma Life*
- Peace & Calming*
- Vetiver
- Cedarwood
- Melissa

Lack of concentration
- Gathering*
- Frankincense
- Vetiver
- Lavender
- Ylang Ylang
- Cedarwood

Racing Heartbeat
- Peace & Calming*
- Stress Away*
- Lavender
- Grounding*
- Ylang Ylang
- Gathering*

Sweating
- Geranium
- Sage
- Peace & Calming*
- Lavender
- Nutmeg
- Clary Sage

Frequent urination or diarrhea
- Digize*
- Fennel
- Copaiba
- Peppermint
- Tea Tree
- Bergamot

Shallow Breathing or unable to catch your breath
- Raven*
- Peppermint
- R.C.*
- Lavender
- Ylang Ylang
- Stress Away*

Dr. B's Top 3 Oils for feeling super anxious:

- Frankincense
- Lavender
- Gathering*

How do I use these oils?:

Again I have listed a lot of oils. I list them because if you happen to have them (or want to buy them) for another reason you can use them for these issues as well. You need to experiment and see what works best for you. For example, some people swear by Peace & Calming while others don't have good results... just experiment. These oils work well blended. I would suggest diffusing two or three that you think would be good together and see if it is helpful. Remember, the best way to get oils to your brain where you need them is to use your hands as diffusers and inhale for 2-3 minutes.

When you are *feeling super anxious* there is an extremely effective way to topically use oils that works great. Have someone put 2-3 drops on your spine... from the top to the bottom. Rub it in! Apply every fifteen minutes or so for one hour. This quickly gets the oils directly into your nervous system. It's a great trick.

Here are the best places to put oils on your body *for when you are feeling super anxious:*
- Spine
- Feet
- Head (all over it!!)
- Heart
- Wrist

Be sure to diffuse a few of your favorite oils 2-3 times a day... and all night!

For Counselors & Helpers.

Sitting with someone who is *feeling super anxious* both takes, and gives energy to me! What about you?

Start your sessions by diffusing *Stress Away* and *Orange*. It smells wonderful and is a great way to reduce the anxious feeling. Make sure you do breathing exercises with your clients each week as you start your time together. Bilateral nostril breathing is one of the best exercises for you to do when your client is feeling anxious (see *All The Stuff* at the end of the book). Have your client put *Lavender*, *Frankincense*, and *Gathering* on their hands before the exercise. If you don't have *Gathering* yet don't worry... just use the other two... they are in your starter kit.

Notes & Oils

CHAPTER 9

TRAUMA SURVIVOR

The impact of trauma has altered our culture. A great working definition of trauma is "anything that is too much, too soon, or too fast for our nervous system to handle, especially if we can't reach a successful resolution." (Banschick, 2015). In reality, it is really hard to pinpoint exactly what events can cause trauma because the experience of trauma is different for everyone. It comes from big events in people's lives that create a *before & after* experience. You were one way *before* the event, and another way *after*.

Although there is a spectrum for the severity of traumatic events, there is no doubt they all change us. They create fear, anxiety, grief, and can shut us down. After living through these times we are often paralyzed and suspicious. Our minds and bodies are put on high alert. It is difficult to engage in our "normal" life. This is because there is no way to go back to "normal" after trauma. Trauma is not just something bad that happens. It is a mind and body altering experience.

Childhood trauma is one of the most difficult things to live through. At my counseling center we use an inventory created by Kaiser Permanente called *The Adverse Childhood Experience Scale (ACE)*. The study of this inventory has shown how childhood trauma has impacted people throughout their lives. The *ACE* has a score between 1-10. In study after study, scoring even a 1 on this scale has been shown to increase the following symptoms by as much as 10 times throughout a lifetime:

- Attempting Suicide
- Heart disease
- Diabetes
- Developmental Delays
- Personality Disorders
- Cancer
- And more...

The effects of trauma on the body are real. Our body stores trauma. If you are interested in reading more about how our bodies store trauma, here are a few books to read:

- *The Body Keeps the Score*
  - author: Bessel van der Kolk, MD. (2015)
- *Waking the Tiger: Healing Trauma*
  - author: Peter Levine (1997)
- *Childhood Disrupted: How your biography becomes your biology, and how you can heal*
  - author: Donna Jackson Nakazawa (2016)

As a therapist I have seen unbelievable amounts of trauma. I have heard stories that have crushed my soul. We have all heard some of these stories. Most of us have lived through them. It is hard to make it through life without experiencing trauma. As a matter of fact, I am not sure it is a good thing for us to never experience trauma in this life. It is true that trauma can forever upset our lives. But it is also true that trauma has the ability to shape us into better people. It causes us to grow and learn. It can give us empathy for others. It puts things into perspective. Traumatic events create a *new normal*.

Symptoms and Impact:

Please note that the symptoms listed here are mostly psychological symptoms of trauma. There is an unending list of physical issues that can happen with trauma as well.

- Intrusive memories of the traumatic event
- Recurrent and distressing dreams related to the event.
- Flashbacks
- Intense reaction to things that remind you of the event.
- Avoiding any situation that might remind you of the event.
- Memory issues
- Low self-esteem
- Lack of confidence
- Shame... a lot of Shame! (Note: Shame is not guilt. Guilt is "I did something bad." Shame is "I am something bad.")
- Intensive negative emotional states (i.e.: fear, anger, guilt)
- Inability to feel positive emotions (i.e.: happiness, joy, loving feelings, satisfaction)
- Irritable

- Anger outbursts
- Self-destructive behavior
- Hypervigilance
- Exaggerated startle response
- Difficulty concentrating
- Difficulty sleeping

Common Treatments:

Counseling*:* Talk therapy has been the way in which counselors traditionally treated symptoms of trauma. However, in recent years, research has shown that it is vital to include *somatic experiences* in therapy. *Somatic experiences* are the feelings we experience in the body. We now know the body stores so much of our trauma. It isn't all just in your head.

Some of the best results for treating trauma come from practitioners who use EMDR (eye movement, desensitization, and reprocessing). This method of therapy helps your brain and body reprocess the trauma in a new way. Incorporating the use of essential oil with EMDR is extremely helpful. The use of oils and therapy together can be amazingly effective!

Another effective way to treat trauma is through a kind of therapy called *Somatic Experiencing.* This involves a lot of body work. Finding a counselor who can work with both your psychological and physiological issues is very important.

No matter what kind of theory or interventions they do, good counselors should also help equip you with skills to use so you can feel better.

Some skills that may help when trauma is messing with your life:

Mindfulness Exercises: There are several mobile apps on your phone that can help you with mindfulness. Mindfulness is just being in the moment. The *here & now* instead of the *there & then.* One of my favorite apps is "Headspace". Check it out.

Breathing Exercises: There are lots and lots of mobile apps to help you with breathing exercises as well. The *Headspace* app has a breathing component. Another app is called "Breathe-Meditation". Some smart watches like the Apple Watch or FitBit will alert you to stop and guide you through brief breathing exercises throughout the day. Check out some of these options and see what you like.

Yoga: Recently there have been several research studies on the impact that yoga has on the results of trauma. I highly recommend this for anyone who has a history of trauma. Find a place that has "trauma informed yoga". It will be one of the best things you can do for yourself.

Progressive Muscle Relaxation: See the instructions in the *All The Stuff* section at the end of the book.

Pharmaceuticals: There are no medications that have specifically been created to help with the results of trauma. However, prescribers will write scripts for a variety of pharmaceuticals which help with the symptoms. Antidepressants and antianxiety medications are prescribed often. Prescribers will also routinely prescribe something to assist with sleep. The side effects to these medications can sometimes be more intrusive than the symptoms. They can, however, be very effective in helping you use therapy more efficiently because they can help clear the "brain fog" that comes after trauma. There are several studies that show that using pharmaceuticals along with therapy increases the effectiveness of both.

Essential Oils for trauma survivors:

Essential oils are highly effective in helping trauma survivors, especially in conjunction with therapy. Essential oils have the ability to tap into both the emotional and memory center of the brain. This can help encourage the processing and release of the trauma. Also, essential oils can help decrease the experience of emotional and physical discomfort. Recent research has found that essential oils can be life changing for war Veterans, helping them have improved sleep, emotional regulation, and more effective relationships. Please know that you don't need to use all of these oils. They are just suggestions. Use one or several. Find what works for you.

Intrusive memories of the traumatic event
- Peace & Calming*
- Vetiver
- SARA*
- Grounding*
- Divine Release*
- Gathering*

Recurrent and distressing dreams related to the event
- Freedom*
- Aroma Sleep*
- Inner Harmony*
- Valor*
- Ylang Ylang
- Gathering*

Flashbacks
- Geranium
- Lavender
- White Angelica
- Grounding*
- Frankincense
- Vetiver

Intense reaction to things that remind you of the event
- Peace & Calming*
- Stress Away*
- Lavender
- Grounding*
- Bergamot
- Hope*

Avoiding situations that remind you of the event
- Peace & Calming*
- Valor*
- Lavender
- Grounding*
- Ylang Ylang
- Gathering*
- SARA*

Memory issues
- Clarity*
- Peppermint
- Rosemary
- Grounding*
- MindWise*
- Vetiver

Low self-esteem
- Bergamot
- Valor*
- Envision*
- Grounding*
- Idaho Blue Spruce
- Rose

Lack of confidence
- Valor
- Bergamot
- frankincense
- Ginger
- Peppermint
- Inner Harmony*

Shame
- Bergamot
- Ylang Ylang
- Frankincense
- Grounding*
- Cedarwood
- Gathering*

Intensive negative emotions & No positive emotions
- Believe*
- Idaho Blue Spruce
- Valor*
- Greatest Potential*
- Trauma Life*
- Tangerine
- SARA*

Irritable & angry outbursts
- Frankincense
- Believe
- Idaho Blue Spruce
- Greatest Potential
- Frankincense
- Bergamot

Hypervigilance
- Vetiver
- Bergamot
- Valor*
- Peace & Calming
- Lavender
- Ylang Ylang

Exaggerated startle response
- Bergamot
- Grounding*
- Sandalwood
- StressAway*
- Ylang Ylang
- White Angelica

Difficulty concentrating
- Gathering*
- Frankincense
- Vetiver
- Lavender
- Ylang Ylang
- Cedarwood

Sleep Disturbance
- Lavender
- Trauma Life
- Peace & Calming
- Frankincense
- Inner Child
- Forgiveness

Dr. B's top 3 oils for Trauma Survivors:
- Gathering*
- SARA*
- Bergamot

How do I use these oils?:

As I have said in other chapters, you need to experiment to find what oils work for you. Experiment with different kinds of applications. The two mistakes most people make are

- Not using enough oil: You need to use several drops… especially at the beginning.
- Not using them often enough: Make sure you are diffusing or applying several times throughout the day.

All of these oils can be diffused and directly applied to your skin.

In one study, veterans with a history of trauma have used *Inner Child* and *Forgiveness* to help with sleep. They have had great results.

Placing oils on the top of your shoulders and the side of your neck is extremely effective for this issue as well.

Here are the best places to put oils on your body *when trauma is messing with you:*

- Spine
- Top of shoulders
- Feet
- Head
- Heart
- Wrist

For Counselors & Helpers:

Vicarious trauma is a real thing. Over time it happens to all counselors. You are not an exception. I know you are strong, resilient, and capable of handling a lot of stuff, but your brain and psyche are still vulnerable. We were not created to handle that much trauma.

In order for you to maintain your effectiveness with people you need to be able to let go of other people's stuff. You need to make sure you are processing all of the things that trigger you through supervision and consultation. You also need to learn how to become aware of when your own sympathetic nervous system becomes activated.

When we are listening to stories of trauma our brains will signal that there is danger. Sometimes our brains don't know it is not our own danger, the information we are hearing just registers as danger. When our brains perceive danger, our sympathetic nervous system becomes activated. I talked about this in the last chapter. Learning to become aware of the triggers that activate your nervous system will help you reduce the amount of vicarious trauma you experience.

When you are working with clients with trauma, here are some tips to try:

- Make sure you are diffusing an oil that will help activate your parasympathetic nervous system. *Bergamot* or *Ylang Ylang* are great for this.
- It can be a good idea to use a diffuser necklace or bracelet when the client needs one oil, but you need another.
- Do breathing exercises during session. This is not just for your client, but for you as well. Breath in *Stress Away* and *Lime* during the exercise.
- Relax your pelvic floor. When you become aware of anxiety in the room, make sure you focus on relaxing your pelvic floor. Your sympathetic nervous system cannot be activated when your pelvic floor muscles are relaxed.
- Belly breathe during session. This also activates your parasympathetic nervous system.
- Above all, focus on self-care throughout your week. Make sure you are doing what you ask your clients to do. (You have got to be *smokin' what you're sellin'.*)

Notes & Oils List

CHAPTER 10
ATTENTION IS NOT MY FORTE

In our culture, paying attention to one thing at a time is nearly impossible. We are constantly being inundated with things to stimulate us. We are always connected (email, texting, social media, etc.). We are given a barrage of things to look at (videos, social media posts). Rather than just *being* and *experiencing* we can't stop doing. This all contributes to our attention difficulties.

I have a hard time paying attention. I didn't always struggle with this but after going to school for a billion years, my ability to pay attention has worn out.

The actual fact is when people, adults and kiddos, have a hard time focusing, it is because their brains can't filter out all of the things around them. If you are like me and have a hard time paying attention, you actually *can't stop* paying attention. I know it sounds counterintuitive, but it's not. Our brains were created to filter out the less important things around us in order to be able to focus on the task at hand. When we can't do that, our focus gets scattered. We can't stop. We go from one thing to another. When we are supposed to be listening to the teacher, we are distracted by the breathing sounds of the person next to us, and the noise of the cars outside, and the light in the hallway... and... and... and...

Another thing that happens is that people with this issue can get, what counselors call, *hyper-focused*. You get stuck. All your focus, and attention, is put in one place. For example, it is difficult to get my attention when I am playing a game on my phone. My family hates it. I can get stuck for hours if I let myself. Nothing can tear me away. People get stuck in a book, on a video game, or movie. Does this sound like anyone you know?

It is hard to be in relationship with someone who struggles with attention and focus. It looks to other people like they are just not trying to focus. If you are the person who can't focus, it can bring up a lot of shame. You want to get stuff done, but then you get stuck. Or you were trying to pay attention to what the person in front of you was saying, but somehow you found yourself thinking about last year's Christmas dinner... then next Christmas dinner... then what am I going to get for dinner tonight. It can be excruciating for everyone.

Homework times with kiddos who struggle with this issue can be a nightmare. Sitting in class, in church, or going to a restaurant, can all be extremely challenging.

Even if you don't struggle with this all the time, there can be times in your life that you are extremely distractible. When your mind is filled with all of the things that are happening in your life, it is hard to focus on the here and now. It is hard to be mindful in the moment. We all struggle with focus. Let's look at some symptoms that happen when this becomes a real issue for people.

Symptoms and Impact:

Here is a list of things that can happen when you have an ongoing struggle with attention.

- Fails to give close attention to details, and makes careless mistakes
- Has a hard time sustaining attention during tasks
- "Staring into space"
- Does not follow through with instructions
- Has a hard time organizing or managing tasks
- Avoids things that call for a sustained mental effort
- Often loses things
- Easily distracted by things around you
- Forgetful in your daily activities

Sometimes people with attention issues can also struggle with the following symptoms:

- Fidgety
- Can't sit still
- Has a hard time relaxing
- "On the go" or "driven by a motor"
- Talk excessively
- Has a hard time waiting
- Often interrupts

Common Treatments:

Counseling: Counseling can help with learning how to focus. Good counselors will be able to give some tricks and skills to learn to manage the way your brain works. If you are feeling distracted and unable to focus because of things in your life that are bothering you, counseling is one of the best ways to work through these things and get back to your old, focused, self.

Some skills that may help with focus & attention:

Mindfulness: Mindfulness skills are the best way to teach your brain to focus. Taking time each day to focus on what is happening in your body is very helpful for people who struggle with focus. Breathing exercises are also extremely helpful. Focusing on your deep breaths, breathing into your belly (not your chest). Feel the breath come in and go out. This will be a life saver. Many other mindfulness exercises are out there for kiddos and adults. Find one that works and do it A LOT!

Practical Tricks:
- Set timers for everything: People who chronically struggle with attention issues have difficulty with the concept of time. It feels like you are going to have to do boring things forever!! Setting a timer will really help maintain focus for short periods of time.
- Don't try to do something for long periods of time without a break. Don't make your kiddo do his homework for an hour... this won't work. Set 5-10 minute timers and give 3

minute breaks. As you can, increase the time they are paying attention.

- Drink caffeine when you need to focus. This seems counterintuitive to give sugar and caffeine to help people pay attention, but if your brain works like most people with this issue, caffeine can help!
- Use essential oils A LOT! This is something I tell all my clients when they need to focus.

Pharmaceuticals: If this is an ongoing issue for you, and you have several of the symptoms as an ongoing concern, then prescribers will consider putting you on a medication that can help. The problem is that the medications for this issue are controlled substances. They are stimulants. These medications are highly addictive. They are also highly effective.

Another concern with this type of medication is that they come with many possible side effects. Make sure that you look into the options. If you are going to use this medication for yourself, or someone you love, add a good routine of essential oils with the medications. This can help balance your body and decrease the side effects that you may experience.

Essential Oils for Focus & Attention:

This section is a much shorter list. I believe that there are a handful of essential oils that are highly effective for attention and focus, and there is no reason to get more. Many of the oils are repeated for each symptom because they work for the overall issue.

NOTE for Kiddos: Although you can use any of these oils for your children, Young Living has a line of oils designed especially for kiddos. The line is called *Kidsents.* GeneYus, one of the best oils you can use for kiddos with a focusing issue, is from that line.

Fails to give close attention to details, and makes careless mistakes
- Vetiver
- Cedarwood
- Lavender
- Focus*
- Peace & Calming*
- Grounding*

Has a hard time sustaining attention during tasks
- Vetiver
- Cedarwood
- Frankincense
- Focus*
- Grounding*
- Gathering*

"Staring into space"
- Vetiver
- Cedarwood
- Myrrh
- Focus*
- Grounding*
- GeneYus*

Does not follow through with instructions
- Vetiver
- Cedarwood
- Ylang Ylang
- Focus*
- Grounding*
- Gathering*

Has a hard time organizing or managing tasks
- Frankincense
- Sandalwood
- Myrrh
- Focus*
- Grounding*
- GeneYus*

Avoids things that call for a sustained mental effort
- Vetiver
- Cedarwood
- Myrrh
- Grounding*
- Gathering*
- GeneYus*

Often loses things
- Vetiver
- Cedarwood
- Lavender
- Focus*
- Peace & Calming*
- Grounding*

Easily distracted by things around you
- Vetiver
- Cedarwood
- Myrrh
- Focus*
- Peace & Calming*
- Grounding*

Forgetful in your daily activities
- Sandalwood
- Ylang Ylang
- Myrrh
- Grounding*
- Gathering*
- GeneYus*

Fidgety
- Lavender
- Frankincense
- Ylang Ylang
- Peace & Calming*
- Grounding*
- GeneYus*

Can't sit still
- Lavender
- Frankincense
- Ylang Ylang
- Focus*
- Peace & Calming*
- Grounding*

Has a hard time relaxing
- Lavender
- Frankincense
- Sandalwood
- Peace & Calming*
- Gathering*
- Valor*

"On the go" or "driven by a motor"
- Vetiver
- Cedarwood
- Lavender
- Focus*
- Peace & Calming*
- GeneYus*

Talk excessively
- Vetiver
- Cedarwood
- Myrrh
- Grounding*
- Gathering*
- Valor*

Has a hard time waiting
- Vetiver
- Frankincense
- Sandalwood
- Peace & Calming*
- Grounding*
- GeneYus*

Often interrupts
- Lavender
- Frankincense
- Ylang Ylang
- Peace & Calming*
- Gathering*
- Valor*

Dr. B's top 3 oils for Trauma Survivors:

- Vetiver
- Cedarwood
- Gathering*

How do I use these oils?:

Using essential oils can have a significant effect in helping with attention and focus because of the effect they have on our limbic system. You want to get them into the limbic system as fast as you can. The best way to do this is to inhale them directly from your hands, put them on the back of your neck, or spine. Re-apply the oils often, especially when you first start using them. It will help balance your body and give you a kick start.

Diffusing these oils can also be really helpful during times that you need to concentrate and focus. Make sure you are doing this often. Two to three times a day!!

For Counselors & Helpers:

My biggest suggestion for working with people who struggle with focus and attention is to diffuse in your office all the time! Try diffusing Lavender and Peppermint. It's a great combo and people love it.

I also suggest if you are having a long day, and struggling to focus on the people in front of you, try using Vetiver and Cedarwood for yourself. Put it on your hands and do some breathing exercises between sessions. This will keep you on top of your game, and able to be present for the people who need you!

Notes & Oils List

CHAPTER 11
THE HEAVY WEIGHT OF ADDICTION

We all know someone who has been affected by the weight of addiction. Actually, if research is right, most of us have experienced some kind of addiction ourselves. Our "drug of choice" could be anything from coffee to heroine. Perhaps your "drug of choice" is work; Maybe it's video games, pornography, or gambling. Whatever you are addicted to can become an anchor in your life. It feels like you can't move without it being right there pulling you down.

Addictions happen for many different reasons. When we are in pain, physically or emotionally, we want to soothe ourselves with something that feels good. Sometimes we just want to be numb, or forget. Sometimes the addiction is exciting. Once our brains get a taste of how fun it can be, we want it all the time.

The problem happens that when we do this over and over, our bodies and brains start to need whatever it is to feel good. We can't feel good without it. As a matter of fact, we start to feel bad without it. Then we begin to need this thing just to make us feel okay. We need it more and more in order to just feel normal.

When people are functioning out of their addiction, it is toxic to relationships. It is said in the counseling world that *the opposite of addiction is connection*. Full blown addiction makes you disconnect from the people around you. This happens for a lot of reasons. Shame, guilt, distraction, avoidance, and many other things get in the way.

Taking the first step is hard. Identifying there is a problem and owning that problem, takes a lot of courage. Then actually doing something to move toward wellness takes plain old hard work.

One of the reasons it is so incredibly hard is that you have no choice but to go through a detox phase. Detoxing from an addiction is not just for smokers, alcoholics, or people with heroin addictions. Detoxing is not only physical, but it taxes you mentally and emotionally. Our brains want our "drug of choice" and will do anything it can to get it. Essential oils can be a huge help in settling your system through the detoxing phase.

Note: It is important to mention that if someone is wanting to detox from alcohol, it must be done while under the supervision of a medical provider.

We all have something that we use to soothe ourselves when we are uncomfortable or stressed. That does not mean it is an addiction. However, if you feel like you can't, or don't know how you would live without it, that can become a problem. Take a deep breath, identify your addiction, and start with baby steps.

Symptoms and Impact:

Here are some things that might be happening if you find yourself under the heavy weight of addiction. If you find yourself saying "yes" to many of these, be sure to talk to someone. Be vulnerable. This is important!

Note: When I talk about your "drug of choice" please know that this is not always a "drug". It can be an activity, or behavior as well (i.e., gambling, pornography, working too much, or even another person).

- There is a significant desire, but with unsuccessful efforts, to cut down or control the use of your "drug of choice"
- A large amount of time is spent in activities necessary to get your "drug of choice"
- Unrelenting cravings and desire for your "drug of choice"
- Failure in fulfilling obligations because of use
- Even though this behavior has caused problems, the use continues
- Give up other activities because of the use
- Even though you know it's hurting you, you still use
- You need more and more in order to get the same feeling
- If you try to stop you experience physical or emotional withdrawals, or both

- People have annoyed you by criticizing the activity or behavior
- You have felt guilty because of the activity or behavior

Common Treatments:

Counseling: It is very helpful to find a person to talk with when you feel the heavy weight of addiction. You need someone who is understanding, empathetic, but who can also hold you accountable. This role is often better suited to someone who is not a friend or family member. People we love have too much invested to be impartial and able to empathize. This is why it is very important to find a good counselor.

Group Therapy: One of the best ways to work through addiction is to find a group. Group therapy has been shown to be the most effective when it comes to overcoming addiction. There are so many groups available (12-step groups like AA or Celebrate Recovery, or alternatives like SMART Recovery, online support groups, etc.). It just takes a first step.

Pharmaceuticals: There are some medications that are made for overcoming specific addictions. There are also medications that are used, by some prescribers, for helping people stop their addictive behavior. Some antianxiety and antidepressant drugs are helpful.

For the most part, people who are trying to overcome addictions do this without medications.

There is always a chance of changing one addiction for another.

Essential Oils for The Heavy Weight of Addiction:

I am not going to list oils by symptoms in this section. These oils will help support your mind and body as you work through the process of letting go of your addiction. If you experience other emotional symptoms, look at the other chapters to identify oils that can help.

Note: Here is a quote from Dr. D. Gary Young's book *Essential Oils Integrative Medical Guide* about addiction:

"Many food and chemical dependencies, such as addictions to tobacco, caffeine, drugs, alcohol, and sugar may originate in the liver. Cleansing and detoxifying the liver is a crucial first step toward breaking free of these addictions.

Trace mineral and mineral deficiencies can also play a part in some addictions. Magnesium, potassium, calcium, and zinc should all be included in the diet." (pg. 270)

Here is a list of essential oils that can help your overall wellness when you are dealing with addiction. Please know that you don't need all of them. Just choose a few and see what works for you.

Single Oils:
- Bergamot
- Black Pepper
- Rosemary
- Vetiver
- Cedarwood
- Lavender
- Grapefruit
- Peppermint
- Clove
- Nutmeg

Oil Blends:
- Peace & Calming
- Grounding
- Tranquil
- Freedom
- Joy
- Forgiveness

Dr. B's top 3 oils for the Heavy Weight of Addiction:
- Tranquil*
- Joy*
- Bergamot

How do I use these oils?:

When you are working on giving up an addiction, your whole focus is on this task. Using essential oils is a good way to change your routine. Use them often, multiple times a day.

Diffuse. Take your diffuser with you. Buy a car diffuser, a diffuser bracelet, and get one for work. Be religious about it.

Directly Inhale: Put a few of your favorite oils in your purse and inhale your "go-to" oil when you start getting cravings. This will help you get past the wave of temptation. Breathe in the oils from your hand for 2-3 minutes at a time. This will get them into your limbic system quickly.

Topically: Put your favorite oils on your neck, spine, and feet. It is also good to put these oils over your heart.

For Counselors & Helpers:

Patience is often hard for me to find when I am working with clients with addictions. It is important to remember addiction is a big deal, even when they don't think it is. Often clients will want to talk about everything else in their life, except the addiction. An accurate assessment of where they are in the "stages of change" is extremely important! It is true that you can work on other things, but keep in mind that it may be to no avail. Working on something else when there is an active addiction is like trying to fix the plumbing when your house is burning down... you can do it, but why? Remember to focus on what is important.

Diffusing bergamot and lavender, or grapefruit and peppermint, would be helpful during session. It would also be so helpful to ask the client if they are willing to do breathing exercises with their favorite oil. It can make all the difference in the world.

Notes & Oils List

ESSENTIALLY BETTER

CHAPTER 12
MEMORIES OF YESTERDAY... BUT NOT TODAY

NOTE: This section has a different outline than all of the others. I am adding this section because it affects so many of us and the people we love. There is very little hope given to us when significant memory issues happen in our brains. Essential oils have potential to be extremely helpful in slowing down the progression of any chronic memory issue. I am adding this section in honor of my mom. I think she is wonderful and deserves to remember how important she is to all who love her.

As I said, I am including this specific issue because it is close to my heart. We all have difficulty remembering things. I can walk from one room to the next and not remember why I was there. I lose my keys weekly, if not daily, and I can't seem to remember anyone's names. Becoming forgetful is part of life. However, sometimes it can become a real problem. When this happens, people begin forgetting how to do familiar tasks and have difficulty keeping up in conversations. They can get very frustrated and agitated because they are unsure what is happening from moment to moment.

Memories from the past seem to become vivid and heightened, but the day to day, moment to moment happenings are never fully in your grasp.

Sometimes there is a need to wander, drive around, walk, or just go anywhere. But there is also an equal need to be home, in a familiar space, able to control your environment.

When memory becomes a real problem in a person's life it is often because they can no longer, or at least with any predictability, put things into their long term memory. It never leaves the short term memory and is lost as soon as it happens. This is why people repeat the same story or question over and over in the same conversation. As soon as it is said, it is gone. It is funny for a while, but then creates fear, anxiety, and frustration for both people in the conversation.

I am excited to list essential oils that have been used to help with memory. There continues to be more and more research on using oils to impact memory. The important thing about using oils for this issue is that they are used very often. This can be hard because the people who need to use them can't remember to do so. Create whatever system you can come up with to encourage consistency of use. This will make or break the success.

Essential Oils for Memory:

Single Oils:
- Rosemary
- Basil
- Peppermint
- Vetiver
- Rose
- Lemon
- Tangerine

Oil Blends:
- Clarity
- Common Sense
- Grounding
- Gathering
- Mindwise
- Peace & Calming
- Tranquil

Dr. B's top 3 oils for the memory:
- Rosemary
- Clarity*
- Common Sense*

How do I use these oils?:

Like I said, the difficulty in using these oils only comes with the ability to remember to use them. If you can create a routine of usage it will really help.

Diffuse or Inhale: Always diffuse Rosemary. This is one of the top oils for supporting our brains and reducing memory loss. Diffuse Common Sense or Clarity as well.

Inhale whatever oils are tolerable. Sometimes this can get a bit agitating. However, most of the time inhaling oils is very welcomed. It is mindful, and makes people experience the moment. The more often you can do this, the more effectiveness you will see.

Make sure to ask what oils they like. Make it a good experience. Then do it over and over. Love on them when you are having them use oils. It will trigger good things in the brain.

What a gift we have to give people who are suffering with memory issues. We have the gift of the moment. Each moment is precious. Make them count.

CHAPTER 13
WRAPPING IT UP

Essential oils make a difference in people's lives. The stories I hear, as well as my own experience, make me a believer. I see and experience change when people begin to use oils for mental and emotional support.

In our culture, toxins are everywhere. Our bodies were not created to handle all of the chemicals that we throw at it every day. When there is a way to decrease the toxins and replace them with natural products, our bodies and brains are much happier. You are worth it. Your family is worth it.

My challenge for you is to work toward wellness. Focus on emotional, mental, and physical wellness for you and your family. Do something intentionally every day to move you closer to your wellness goals.

Give yourself grace. Use your oils. Share them with a friend.

Starting from the beginning?

Are you interested in using essential oils for yourself, your family, or people you work with and wondering where to start? The best way to get started is to invest in a premium starter kit with Young Living. This kit gives you a well-rounded set of oils that will be helpful for every aspect of your life... and it comes with a diffuser!!! Once you purchase your starter kit you are then able to buy products from Young Living at the wholesale price!

Here's how to get started:

If someone gave you this book, ask them how to get started. They will help you through the process!!

If not, I would love to have you in my group of people getting *Essentially Better*.

Here's what you do...

- Go to http://yl.pe/78pb
- Choose a membership & continue
- Choose a starter kit & check out
- Wait patiently for your kit to arrive
- Open your box and start your journey!

Note: As part of my Young Living group you will receive a monthly newsletter from me. We have a great, supportive team!

ALL THE STUFF

Square Breathing:

This is used to calm down your heart rate and activate your parasympathetic nervous system (that's a good thing)!

- Sit in a chair with both your feet on the floor.
- Breath in (through your nose) for four counts... 1,2,3,4
- Hold your breath for four counts... 1,2,3,4
- Breath out (through your mouth) for four counts... 1,2,3,4
- Hold for four counts... 1,2,3,4
- Repeat this four times.

Try to breathe so deeply that your belly rises on the in breath and deflates like a balloon on the out breath.

Note: Use a variety of essential oils with this technique... place 2-6 drops of oils on your hand and use the hand diffuser method throughout this exercise.

Alternate (Bilateral) Nostril Breathing:

Reference & Credit: This is directly taken from the following website: **https://chopra.com**

Next time you find yourself doing too many things at once, or you sense panic or anxiety begin to rise, move through a few rounds of alternate nostril breathing. It's a great way to hit the reset button for your mental state.

- Take a comfortable and tall seat, making sure your spine is straight and your heart is open.
- Relax your left palm comfortably into your lap and bring your right hand just in front of your face.
- With your right hand, bring your pointer finger and middle finger to rest between your eyebrows, lightly using them as an anchor. The fingers we'll be actively using are the thumb and ring finger.
- Close your eyes and take a deep breath in and out through your nose.
- Close your right nostril with your right thumb. Inhale through the left nostril slowly and steadily.
- Close the left nostril with your ring finger so both nostrils are held closed; retain your breath at the top of the inhale for a brief pause.
- Open your right nostril and release the breath slowly through the right side; pause briefly at the bottom of the exhale.
- Inhale through the right side slowly.
- Hold both nostrils closed (with ring finger and thumb).
- Open your left nostril and release breath slowly through the left side. Pause briefly at the bottom.
- Repeat 5-10 cycles, allowing your mind to follow your inhales and exhales.

Steps 5-9 represent one complete cycle of alternate nostril breathing. If you're moving through the sequence slowly, one cycle should take you about 30-40 seconds. Move through 5-10 cycles when you're feeling stressed, anxious, or in need of a reset button.

Tip: Consistency is helpful, so try to match the length of your inhales, pauses, and exhales. For example, you can start to inhale for a count of five, hold for five, exhale for five, hold for five. You can slowly increase your count as you refine your practice.

Sleep Hygiene Protocol:

This is a sleep protocol that is helpful for some people.

Reference & Credit: This is taken from the DBT skills training handouts and worksheets, **second edition** by Marsha M. Linehan (emotion regulation handout 20b).

To increase the likelihood of restfulness/sleep:

- **Develop and follow a consistent sleep schedule, even on weekends.** Go to bed and get up at the same times each day, and avoid anything longer than a 10-minute nap during the day.
- **Do not use your bed in the daytime** for things like watching tv, talking on the phone, or reading.
- **Avoid** caffeine, nicotine, alcohol, heavy meals, and exercise late in the day before going to sleep.
- **When preparing to sleep, turn off the light, keep the room quiet and the**

temperature comfortable and relatively cool. Try an electric blanket if you are cold; putting your feet outside of the blanket or turning on a fan directed toward your bed if you are hot; or wearing a sleeping mask, using earplugs, or turning on a 'white noise' machine if needed.

- **Give yourself half an hour to at most an hour to fall asleep.** If it doesn't work, evaluate whether you are calm, or anxious (even if only "background anxiety"), or ruminating.

- **Do not catastrophize.** Remind yourself that you need rest, and aim for relaxation (i.e., dreaminess) and resting your brain. Sell yourself on the idea that staying awake is not a catastrophe. Do not decide to give up on sleeping for the night and get up for the "day".

If you are calm but wide awake:

- **Get out of bed; go to another room and read a book** or do some other activity that will not wake you up further. As you begin to get tired and/or sleepy, go back to bed.
- **Try a light snack** (e.g., an apple)

If you are anxious or ruminating:

- **Put really cold water on your face. Get right back in bed and do some square breathing.** Remember, if you have any medical condition, get medical approval before using cold water.

- **Try the 9-0 mindfulness practice.** Breathe in deeply and breathe out slowly, saying in your mind the number 9. On the next breath out, say 8; then say 7, and so on until you breathe out saying 0. Then start over, but this time start with 8 (instead of 9) as you breathe out, followed by 7, and so on until you reach 0. Next start with 7 (instead of 8) as you breathe out, followed by 6. Next, start with 6 as you breathe out, and so on to 0. Then start with 5, then with 4, and so on until you have gone all the way down to starting with 1. (If you get lost, start over with the last number you remember.) Continue until you fall asleep.

- **Focus on bodily sensations** of the rumination. (Rumination is often an escape from difficult emotional sensations.)

- **Reassure yourself** that worries in the middle of the night are just 'middle-of-the-night thinking,' and that in the morning you will think and feel differently.

- **Read an emotionally engrossing novel** for a few minutes until you feel somewhat tired. Then stop reading, close your eyes, and try to continue the novel in your head.

- **If rumination doesn't stop, follow these guidelines:** If it's solvable, solve it. If it is insolvable, plan a time for the next day to experience feelings about being out of control.

If nothing else works, with eyes closed, listen to public radio at a low volume (use headphones if necessary). Public radio is a good choice for this because there is little fluctuation in voice tone or volume.

Progressive Muscle Relaxation:

STEP ONE: Tension

The first step is applying muscle tension to a specific part of the body. First, focus on the target muscle group, for example, your left hand. Next, take a slow, deep breath and squeeze the muscles as hard as you can for about 5 seconds. Try to ONLY tense the muscles you are targeting. Isolating muscle groups gets easier with practice.

STEP TWO: Relaxing the Tense Muscles

This step involves quickly relaxing the tensed muscles. After about 5 seconds, let all the tightness flow out of the tensed muscles. Exhale as you do this step. It is important to very deliberately focus on and notice the difference between the tension and relaxation. This is the most important part of the whole exercise.

Remain in this relaxed state for about 15 seconds, and then move on to the next muscle group. Repeat the tension-relaxation steps.

Start with your feet and systematically move up

- Foot (curl your toes downward)
- Lower leg and foot (tighten your calf muscle by pulling toes towards you)
- Entire leg (squeeze thigh muscles while doing above)

(Repeat on other side of body)

- Hand (clench your fist)
- Entire right arm (tighten your biceps by drawing your forearm up towards your

shoulder and "make a muscle", while clenching fist)
(Repeat on other side of body)

- Buttocks
- Stomach
- Chest
- Neck and shoulders (raise your shoulders up to touch your ears)
- Mouth (open your mouth wide enough to stretch the hinges of your jaw)
- Eyes (clench your eyelids tightly shut)
- Forehead (raise your eyebrows as far as you can)

It can be helpful to listen to someone guide you through these steps. There are many relaxation apps, or free online videos, available that will take you through a progressive muscle relaxation.

Thinking Errors that Trigger Anxiety:

This information was taken from a blog on Psychology Today's Website, *10 Thinking Errors that will Crush Your Mental Strength: and how to overcome them.* These are common thinking errors. Check out the blog for great ideas on how to change the way you think and overcome these anxiety triggers.

1. **All-or-Nothing Thinking:** Seeing things as good or bad, black or white, right or wrong.

2. **Overgeneralizing:** Taking one situation or incident and applying it to your whole life, or to "every time".

3. **Filtering Out the Positive:** When nine good things happen, and one bad thing, we focus on the bad. When someone says nine good things about you and one criticism, you hold onto the criticism as truth.

4. **Mind-Reading:** This is when we think we can be sure what someone else is thinking. We assumes we know what's going on in someone else's mind. "He must have thought I was stupid."

5. **Catastrophizing:** This is when we assume we will end up in the worst possible situation. "I have a headache, I'm probably going to die!"

6. **Emotional Reasoning:** This is assuming that our emotions are always based on reality. (FYI... they aren't!!)

7. **Labeling:** Labeling is putting a name to something. Instead of thinking, "He made a mistake," you might label your husband as "an idiot."

8. **Fortune-telling:** This is assuming we know the future. Saying things to yourself like "I am going to hate going to that party!" or "This is going to be an awful day!"

9. **Personalization:** It's easy to make everything about us. This is when you think that other people's actions are always about your. If a friend doesn't call you, you assume, "I knew it... she's mad at me."

10. **Unreal Ideal:** Making unfair comparisons about ourselves and other people. Thinking you should be somewhere in life that you are not.

Wellness Planning Handout:

I use this handout for a workshop I do on holistic wellness planning. This workshop is very helpful for people who have started to use oils for emotional support and want to begin a more holistic approach to using oils.

Feel free to use this, change it any way you want, and share it with your friends.

Essential Oils & Wellness Planning Workshop Handout
~your wellness journey begins here~

This is a short (can you believe it's short) list of some oils and supplements that will help support each different area of wellness. This is by no means an exhaustive list. This is just something to help you get an idea of how oils might be used to support every system in your body. Essential oils are created with complex molecules. (Ok...don't tune out because of the "science nerd" words.) This means with just one oil you can support several different systems in your body. We are created to be integrated and whole beings... We are beautifully and wonderfully made!!

Take a look...

Disclaimer:
PLEASE NOTE: The oils that are suggested here are to support your body's wellness. I am in no way suggesting that essential oils can cure disease or disorders.

Physical Wellness
Systems of the body:

Vascular System: Circulation, heart, arteries, veins: delivers oxygen and nutrients to organs and cells
- **Oils:**
  - Circulation blend:
    - 6 drops of lavender
    - 4 drops of rosemary
    - 2 drops vetiver or jasmine
    - 1 oz carrier oil
  - Peppermint!! Supports circulation
  - Geranium Rose

- **Supplements:**
  - Ningxia Red

Digestive System: mouth esophagus, stomach, intestines: mechanical and chemical processes that provide nutrients, eliminate waste from the body.
- **Oils:**
  - Digestive blend
    - 3 drops Roman Chamomile
    - 3 drops lemongrass
    - 2 drops ginger
    - 2 drops peppermint
    - Carrier oil
  - Digize
  - Peppermint
  - Frankincense
  - Lemon
  - Tea Tree & Oregano
  - Fennel
- **Supplements:**
  - **Ningxia** Red
  - Digest & Cleanse
  - ComforTone Capsules ~ Cleanse... promotes liver, gall bladder, stomach health
  - ICP 8 oz ~ Helps keep your colon clean... fiber that scours out residues.

Endocrine System: Hormones: Provides chemical communications within the body
- **Oils:**
  - Happy Mama Blend:
    - 5 drops lavender
    - 3 drops clary sage
    - 1 drop ylang ylang
    - carrier oil
  - EndoFlex
  - Clary Sage

- o Progessence Plus~ helps with low libido, PMS, endometriosis, PCOS, fibromyalgia, hot flashes, infertility, mood swings, weight control (2 drops on neck once a day
- o Dragon Time~ PMS
- o Ylang Ylang~ Helps balance anger, filter negative energy
- o Spearmint~ balances thyroid hormones
- o Myrtle~ thyroid hormones
- o Nutmeg~ supports adrenal glands
- o German chamomile~ protects liver
- o Geranium~ balances hormones
- o Sage~ strengthens vital organs
- o For Men:
- o Shutran
- o Mister
- **Supplements:**
  - o **Ningxia**
  - o Helpful for Adrenal Fatigue:
    - Super C
    - Thyromin
    - Super B

Exocrine System: Skin, hair, nails, sweat glands
- **Oils:**
  - o Frankincense
  - o Lavender
  - o Citronella (acne, eczema)
  - o Tea Tree
- **Supplements:**
  - o **Ningxia**
  - o Sulfurzyme~ Helps maintain the structure of proteins

Immune / Lymphatic System: lymph nodes: defends the body against pathogenic viruses that may endanger the body
- **Oils:**
  - o Immune Support Blend

- 10 drops Frankincense
- 20 drops Thieves
- 20 drops Lemon
- 10 drops Peppermint
- carrier oil
  - Rosemary
  - Clove
  - Eucalyptus
  - Cinnamon
  - Wild Orange
- **Supplements:**
  - **Ningxia**
  - Inner Defense
  - ImmuPro

Muscular System: muscles: enables the body to move
- **Oils:**
  - "Pain in the..." Blend
    - 10 drops Copaiba
    - 10 drops Panaway
    - 10 drops Valor
    - carrier oil
  - Panaway
  - Wintergreen
  - Copaiba
  - Valor
  - Citronella (muscle pain, nerve pain)
  - Ginger (with copaiba and wintergreen)

Nervous System: Collects and processes information from the senses via nerves and the brain and tells us what to do and what to feel.
- **Oils:**
  - Nerve Pain Blend:
    - 4 drops chamomile
    - 3 drops helichrysum
    - 2 drops lavender

- 3 drops marjoram
- 1 oz carrier oil
  - Helichrysum
  - Peppermint
  - Wintergreen
  - Geranium Rose
  - Eucalyptus
  - Rosemary

Renal/Urinary System: kidneys: filter the blood
- **Oils:**
  - Bladder Trouble Blend (put over bladder & take with Ningxia)
    - 3 drops Frankincense
    - 3 drops Thieves
    - 3 drops Lemon
  - Melrose
  - Sage
  - Immupower
  - Bergamot
- **Supplements:**
  - **Ningxia**
  - Inner Defense
  - AlkaLime
  - ImmuPro

Reproductive System: sexual organs: reproduction and sexuality (GET "LUCY LIBIDO" Best book on this subject!!)
- **Oils:**
  - FOR CRAMPS: 2 drops Panaway + carrier oil. Then add 2 drops peppermint and rub on lower abdomen and back
  - SclarEssence
  - Ylang Ylang
  - Lavender
  - Eucalyptus
  - Rose

- ○ Support for PCOS (Polycystic Ovarian Syndrome)
    - ▪ Geranium
    - ▪ Rose
    - ▪ Fennel
    - ▪ Clary Sage

Respiratory System: lungs, trachea: bring air into and out of the body.
- **Oils:**
    - ○ Breathe Again Roll on
    - ○ RC
    - ○ Raven
    - ○ Lemon, Lavender, Peppermint!!!!
    - ○ Eucalyptus

Skeletal System: Bones, ligaments: supports the body and its organs
- **Oils:**
    - ○ Deep Relief Roll-on
    - ○ RC (for bone spurs)
    - ○ Wintergreen
- **Supplements:**
    - ○ **Ningxia**
    - ○ BLM

Overall Physical Wellness:

Weight and Nutrition
- ○ Slique: This whole line is created to support weight loss
- ○ Peppermint
- ○ Any Citrus oils

Sleep
- ○ Trauma Life
- ○ Sleep Essence
- ○ Peace & Calming
- ○ Stress Away
- ○ Lavender

- o Vetiver
- o Bergamot

Pain

- o Panaway
- o M Grain
- o Aroma Siez
- o Peppermint

Exercise

- o Motivation
- o All Supplements

Emotional Wellness
Emotional Regulation/ Distress Tolerance

Anxiety

- o "Chill Out" Blend
  - ▪ 5 drops Vetiver
  - ▪ 5 drops Lavender
  - ▪ 5 drops Stress Away
  - ▪ 5 drops Joy
  - ▪ 5 drops Valor II
  - ▪ Carrier Oil
- o Peace & Calming
- o Bergamot
- o Cedarwood
- o Tons of others...

Sadness

- o Bergamont
- o Clary Sage
- o Frankincense
- o Orange
- o Ylang Ylang
- o Trauma Life
- o Stress Away
- o Hope

- Envision

Anger

- Bergamot
- Patchouli
- Roman Chamomile
- Rose
- Vetiver
- Ylang Ylang

Lack of Confidence/Self-Esteem

- Valor
- Valor II
- Bergamot
- Grapefruit
- Jasmine
- Orange
- Rosemary

Spirituality

Oils to support spiritual growth:

- **Surrender**
  Surrender is a great oil for prayer, yoga, letting go of hurt feelings... etc.
- **Hope**
  This oil makes me cry sometimes... it is one of my favorites
- **Acceptance**
  Promotes focus during prayer and meditation, often used in yoga.
- **Frankincense**
  Used in prayer time throughout time.

Relational

Oola Blends

- **Family**
  Supports the development of love, patience, respect
- **Finances**
  Supports the development abundance and clarity
- **Faith**
  Supports the development of spiritual awareness
- **Fun**
  Boosts self-confidence and positivity
- **Fitness**
  Uplifts, inspires and energizes
- **Friends**
  Supports the development of self-confidence and self-worth
- **Field**
  Supports the development self-worth and strength
- **Balance**
  Helps focus on passions and behaviors
- **Grow**
  Promotes courage and progress

Patience

- **"Mama's Morning" Blend**
  - 12 drops tangerine
  - 4 drops lavender
  - 4 drops ylang ylang
  - 4 drops peppermint

Environmental Wellness

Cleaning Products

- Thieves Cleaning products

Hygiene Products

- Shampoo & conditioner
- Toothpaste
- Mouthwash

Makeup/Facial products
- ○ Savvy Minerals
- ○ ART
- ○ Lip balm
- ○ Orange Blossom Facial Wash

Wellness Planning Worksheet:

I use this at our *Wellness Planning* Workshops, and when I am working with someone who wants to make a wellness plan for a holistic approach to essential oils.

Feel free to use this, change it any way you want, and share it with your friends.

Essential Oils & Wellness
Planning Worksheet

Overall Wellness Goals:

What are your overall wellness goals... for yourself and your family... think holistically... body, mind, spirit?

Now let's get specific:

Physical Wellness:

- For what things would you like to use essential oils instead of over the counter products?
- What pharmaceuticals do you use that could be supported by essential oils?
- What systems of your body could be better supported by using essential oils?
- Do you have concerns with your
  - _____ Weight
  - _____ Sleep
  - _____ Nutrition (what you eat)
  - _____ Pain
  - _____ Exercise

Emotional & Mental Wellness

- How does anxiety or depression impact your life?
- How skillful are you in regulating your moods? (Use a scale of 1-10.)
- When do you struggle with focusing on the present moment or what you are doing?
- What are the specific things regarding your emotional and mental wellness you would like to focus on this year using essential oils?

Spiritual Wellness:

- What specific areas of your spiritual life would you like to focus on in the next several months?
- What are you holding onto from your past or present that you would like to be able to surrender?
- Are there things in your life that you have hoped for and now you feel resigned that they will never happen? What are they?

Relational Wellness

- What are specific relational concerns that you would like to work on this year?
- How have you practiced forgiveness? Is this difficult?
- Where do you wish you had more energy in/for your relationships?

Environmental Wellness

What chemical based products do you use that could be changed out for natural products?

Prioritize

You can do it all... just not all at once!

What do you want to work on over...
- the next month?
- the next 3 months?
- the next 6 months?

Emotional Wellness Blends:

ESSENTIAL OIL BLEND RECIPES SUGGESTIONS
FROM D. GARY YOUNG
(for rollerballs add fractionated coconut oil)

Energy Blend (From Gary Young's Essential Oils Integrative Medical Guide pg. 180) • 40 drops rosemary • 30 drops balsam fir • 20 drops juniper • 10 drops nutmeg • 10 drops pepper • 3 drops blue tansy	*Clarity Blend* (From D. Gary Young's Essential Oils Integrative Medical Guide pg. 176) • 40 drops cardamom • 30 drops rosemary • 10 drops vetiver • 5 drops peppermint • 5 drops geranium • 3 drops basil
Emotional Release Blend (From D. Gary Young's Essential Oils Integrative Medical Guide pg. 179) • 20 drops German Chamomile • 10 drops ledum • 30 drops ylang ylang • 25 drops geranium • 15 drops sandalwood	*Abuse Blend* (From D. Gary Young's Essential Oils Integrative Medical Guide pg. 165) • 40 drops ylang ylang • 30 drops geranium • 20 drops lavender • 10 drops cedarwood • 15 drops balsam fir • 5 drops rose • 16 drops orange • 4 drops helichrysum

(Young, 2003)

MORE ESSENTIAL OIL BLEND RECIPES

(for rollerballs add fractionated coconut oil)

CIRCULATION lavender, vetiver, rosemary (or purification)	**LUCY LIBIDO** clary sage, bergamot, lavender, release
TUMMY digize, peppermint, wintergreen, copaiba	**BREATHE** RC, eucalyptus, peppermint, purification
HAPPY MAMMA lavender, clary sage, ylang ylang, joy	**SLEEP** trauma life, peace & calming, lavender
SKIN Lavender, frankincense, tea tree	**OH MY HEAD** m-grain, aroma size, peppermint
IMMUNE (Wellness) frankincense, thieves, lemon, peppermint	**RELAX** vetiver, lavender, stress away, joy, valor
PAIN IN THE... copaiba, panaway, valor	**PRAY** sacred frankincense, hope, vetiver
NERVES lavender, eucalyptus, wintergreen	**MAMA'S MORNING** tangerine, lavender, ylang ylang, peppermint
BLADDER TROUBLE frankincense, thieves, lemon.	**THIEVES CLEANER** Thieves cleaner and water.
FOCUS cedarwood, lavender, vetiver	**ZEN** frankincense, lavender, bergamot
SNIFFLES lemon, lavender, peppermint	**CHILL / CALM** frankincense, stress away, lavender, copaiba
ENERGY lemon, eucalyptus, peppermint cinnamon	**ENERGY** (second option) grapefruit, rosemary, peppermint

ESSENTIALLY BETTER

REFERENCE LIST

Adverse Childhood Experiences Scale. (2006, October24).Retrieved February 1, 2018 from https://www.ncjfcj.org/sites/default/files/Finding%20Your%20ACE%20Score.pdf.

American Psychiatric Association. (2013). Diagnostic and statistical manual of mental disorders : **DSM-5** (5th ed.). Arlington, VA: American Psychiatric Association.

Banschick, M. (2015, May 3). Somatic experiencing: how trauma can be overcome [Web log post]. Retrieved February 2, 2018, from https://www.psychologytoday.com

Linehan, M. (2014) *DBT skills training manual: 2nd edition.* New York, NY: The Guilford Press.

Morin, A. (2015, January, 24). 10 Thinking errors that will crush your mental strength... and how to overcome them [Web log post]. Retrieved February 12, 2018, from https://www.psychologytoday.com

Worwood, V.A. (2016) *The Complete Book if Essential Oils and Aromatherapy*. United Kingdom: New World Library.

Young, D.G. (2003) *Essential Oils Integrative Medical Guide: Building Immunity, Increasing Longevity, and Enhancing Mental Performance with Therapeutic-Grade Essential Oils*. Lehi, UT: Life Sciences Press.

ABOUT THE AUTHOR

Dr. Wendy Bruton is a licensed professional counselor. She is the owner and executive director of *The Soul Care Center* in Salem, OR. The Soul Care Center provides holistic mental health services including counseling, aromatherapy, yoga, massage, and hypnotherapy.

Dr. Bruton is a counselor educator and has taught at several universities around the country. She is also a sought after speakers and consultant for businesses regarding mental health and wellness.

She is married to Scott, her high school sweetheart. They have four children, and four grandchildren.

If you would like to contact Dr. Bruton for speaking or consultation scheduling, please contact her at

oilsforfeelings@gmail.com

Made in the USA
Columbia, SC
06 July 2020

12145830R00078